Health Care in Transition

Technology Assessment in the Private Sector

Richard A. Rettig

Supported by the

Department of
Health and Human Services

Office of the Assistant Secretary for
Planning and Evaluation/Health

Agency for
Health Care Policy and Research

*Critical
Technologies
Institute*

and

*Health Sciences
Program*

RAND

Medical technology, broadly construed, embraces all innovations in medicine—new drugs, biologics, medical devices, and procedures— as well as existing therapeutic and diagnostic capabilities. The evaluation of the clinical effectiveness and cost-effectiveness of medical technology, therefore, is a matter of substantial interest to many parties. *Technology assessment* (TA) is the term most often applied to such evaluation.

Much attention has been given in the past two decades to the exercise of a strong federal government role in technology assessment, most notably with the creation of the National Center for Health Care Technology (NCHCT) within the Public Health Service in the late 1970s. Discontinued in 1982, NCHCT was succeeded by a smaller Office of Health Technology Assessment (OHTA). When NCHCT met its demise, policymakers turned to nongovernment or public-private alternatives, one of which was the Council on Health Care Technology of the Institute of Medicine, which existed from 1985 through 1989. Another alternative was proposed by the Physician Payment Review Commission in 1994: a new government agency for national coverage decisions. Both of these entities, one actual and one proposed, were national or centralized organizations.

A strong national TA organization has not developed, however, either at the federal government level or in the private sector, and it appears unlikely that the situation will change any time in the near future. From the perspective of the 1993–1994 failure of health-care-reform legislation, the forceful emergence of managed care, and the continuing rapid change in all aspects of the health care system, questions arise about the extent of TA activity in the private health care sector, especially in managed care: Does this activity fulfill the functions that were once expected of the federal government? What are the implications of these developments for the federal government's role in TA? These questions are the subject of this report.

This report is addressed to all those concerned with the institutions and processes by which medical technology is evaluated, both in the public and private sectors of the health care system. Those concerned with clinical practice guidelines will also find the report of interest, because both TA and guidelines share a commitment to evidence-based analyses. The audience for this report includes not just those having focused responsibilities in technology assessment, but all those policymakers and managers who are actual or prospective users of TA. In the federal government, the audience includes members of Congress and their staff, and officials in the Department of Health and Human Services, the Department of Veterans Affairs, and the Department of Defense. In state governments, Medicaid programs and health insurance commissioners should also find it useful. The private-sector audience includes managed care organizations, health insurance companies, indemnity insurers, corporate purchasers of health care services, health-insurance-purchasing cooperatives, hospitals, physicians, and manufacturers of drugs, biologics, and medical devices.

The research for this report was sponsored by the Office of the Assistant Secretary for Planning and Evaluation/Health (ASPE) and the Agency for Health Care Policy and Research (AHCPR), both of the Department of Health and Human Services. Publication of this report was supported by Research Staff Management Department (RSMD) funds. This report is based on research conducted under the auspices of RAND's Critical Technologies Institute and Health Sciences program.

CONTENTS

TABLES

INTRODUCTION

Medical technology, broadly construed, embraces all innovations in medicine—new drugs, biologics, medical devices, and procedures—as well as existing therapeutic and diagnostic capabilities. The evaluation of the clinical effectiveness and cost-effectiveness of medical technology, therefore, is a matter of substantial interest to many parties. *Technology assessment* (TA) is the term most often applied to such evaluation.

Innovation in medical technology has been identified by many analysts as a major factor driving the relentless increase in national expenditures for health care services. At the same time, innovation in medicine is regarded by many as a primary guarantor of quality health care and the only pathway to finding new solutions to both old and new clinical problems.

The efforts, largely unsuccessful, to establish a national technology-assessment capability in the federal government, or in the nonprofit sector, reveal this deeply rooted societal ambivalence toward medical technology—the wish to control health care costs, but not at the expense of innovation, quality, and clinical progress. Society, however, is not a decisionmaker, and societal ambivalence toward TA is seldom found at the level of the interested parties. Indeed, political opposition to TA by those developing and bringing to market new health and medical care products has been expressed strongly and effectively for over two decades.

However, the health-system environment in which TA is performed
has changed profoundly in the past five years. The failure to enact
federal health-care-reform legislation in 1994 both diminished the
role of the federal government and released private-sector energies.
Large corporate purchasers of health care have become more active
in seeking to rein in the growth of health care expenditures.
Managed care organizations have responded to market opportunities by enrolling an increasing proportion of patients, reducing ex-
cess hospital capacity, and shifting care away from physician specialists to primary caregivers.

In this context, the evaluation of medical practice—mainly for *clinical effectiveness* (what works in day-to-day practice) but also for cost-
effectiveness—has assumed greater market value. In short, the demand for TA and other forms of evaluation has increased.
Traditional forms of medical-technology evaluation that occur at the
beginning of the innovation process include Food and Drug
Administration (FDA) evaluation of drugs and medical devices for
safety and *efficacy* (what works under carefully controlled conditions) and clinical trials for evaluating the efficacy of medical
procedures. Among more-recent means of evaluation, technology
assessment occurs after the FDA decision, mainly at the boundary
between the introduction of a new medical technology and the
decision to reimburse it. Clinical practice guidelines, by contrast,
come into play for widely accepted, although not always well-
evaluated, clinical practices. Both TA and practice guidelines draw
heavily on health services research about efficacy, effectiveness, *outcomes* (the benefits of clinical intervention for populations or individual patients), and *appropriateness* (the benefits of an effective intervention when used for a specific patient).

PERFORMERS OF TECHNOLOGY ASSESSMENT

Historically, the policy discussion of technology assessment has focused mainly on the role of the federal government. This report
briefly describes a number of private-sector health organizations that
are engaged today in technology assessment—the performers of TA.
This information is not a comprehensive enumeration of *all* such organizations but a selective picture of the *major* ones, including several national TA subscription services. Some national insurers

and/or managed care organizations conduct centralized TA that serves member plans. Several membership organizations have constituency-oriented TA programs. And some individual managed care organizations have significant TA capability. In short, the private-sector TA "system" is a mix of centralized (national subscription, plan, and constituency efforts) and decentralized (regional and local health plan efforts) activities.

This report emphasizes managed care organizations—traditional group- and staff-model health maintenance organizations (HMOs) or more loosely organized preferred provider organizations (PPOs), independent practice associations (IPAs), or mixed models. In all these forms of managed care, physicians are placed at financial risk either by capitation or by discounting of fees. There are three reasons for this emphasis in the report. First, managed care constitutes the most visible and rapidly changing element in a changing health care system, and it deserves attention for that reason alone. Second, the incentives of managed care to limit the provision of medical services place a premium on knowing what medical care is effective. Thus, there is reason to believe that TA might be more highly valued in managed care than in fee-for-service medicine.

Third, it is appropriate—in the mid-1990s—to move beyond undifferentiated studies of all those engaged in TA to sector analyses—of hospitals, physicians, insurers/managed care, and the therapeutic products industries (pharmaceutical, biotechnology, medical device). Each sector differs in its incentives to develop and use medical technology; therefore, incentives to support or conduct technology assessment differ correspondingly. It appears from the evidence in this report that managed care has strong incentives to support and conduct TA in the current environment.

THE CONTENT OF TECHNOLOGY ASSESSMENT

This report examines the content of TA, which is characterized by major analytical and methodological strategies, with respect to its changing scope (e.g., more attention is being given to the evaluation of new drugs than before, and sole reliance upon FDA approval is less frequent). Most important, a strong conceptual and methodological development within TA has been the movement toward *evidence-based medicine.* Through rigorous and systematic review of the scientific literature, this movement seeks to develop a strong scientific base for what is known about effective clinical practice.

Although consensus processes that rely on experts and other interested parties are still used to interpret and apply the results of TAs, the exclusive use of such processes to *establish* the scientific bases of clinical practice is heavily discounted, unless it is preceded by rigorous analyses of the scientific evidence. Methodologically, priority-setting processes are well developed in the private sector and are unencumbered by the administrative procedures required by federal agencies; cost-effectiveness analysis is on the verge of being used in decisionmaking; TA and clinical practice guidelines show substantial convergence (although the former focuses more on specific technologies and procedures, and the latter focuses on the management of clinical problems or disease conditions); and the need for greater attention to improved design and conduct of clinical trials is increasingly clear.

THE USES OF THE RESULTS OF TECHNOLOGY ASSESSMENT

Technology assessment in the managed care sector primarily supports coverage decisionmaking. However, a number of innovative developments go beyond the narrow range of issues encompassed by such decisionmaking. They include benchmarking, for member organizations, of evaluative activities believed to be needed for survival in the current marketplace; providing a forum for reviewing the evidence related to competing technologies; allowing experimentation on "roll out" (diffusion) strategies for the rational introduction of new technologies; and offering education directed at changing physician behavior toward evidence-based medicine.

IMPLICATIONS FOR PUBLIC-PRIVATE RELATIONSHIPS

Finally, an examination of private-sector TA leads back to questions about the appropriate role of the federal government in TA and the appropriate division of labor between the public and private sectors. One strong implication is that the federal government as a purchaser of health care services should be no less competent and effective than the private sector in its support and conduct of TA. However, this does not necessarily imply a centralized federal government leadership role, which does not appear politically feasible at present. Another implication is that both public and private sectors should emphasize the use of evidence-based assessments and the further development of cost-effectiveness as operational tools. In addition, as evidence-based assessments reveal the weaknesses of the clinical literature, the need becomes clearer for a feedback loop from TA performers to the organizations that sponsor and perform clinical trials.

Both sectors should also promote the convergence of technology assessment and clinical practice guidelines. These activities have some differences but share a commitment to evidence-based medicine and have common methodologies. The effective use of TA beyond coverage decisionmaking should also be promoted. Finally, among the various forms of public and private cooperation, the sponsorship of TA-related research remains a distinct role for the federal government. Such research generates benefits available to all and is extremely modest in cost relative to the benefits received.

ACKNOWLEDGMENTS

Two veterans of technology assessment discussions, Cheryl Austein, Director of the Division of Public Health Policy of the Office of the Assistant Secretary for Planning and Evaluation/Health (ASPE), and Peter Bouxsein, then Assistant to the Administrator of the Agency for Health Care Policy and Research (AHCPR), served as project officers. They supplied a continuing reality test throughout the project. The report benefited greatly from an internal RAND review by Elizabeth McGlynn and from the editorial discipline of Marian Branch and Miriam Polon.

Chapter One

INTRODUCTION

HEALTH CARE IN TRANSITION

The U.S. health care system is changing in practically all dimensions. Change is occurring at the level of the nation's health *system*, within all *major elements* of the system, and in the established *relationships* among elements of the system. Elements that were once loosely coupled are now being drawn into tighter relationships. Important changes include the following:

- Large corporate purchasers of health care have become increasingly aggressive in seeking to reduce the costs of health care that they bear, and, concurrently, are focusing explicitly on the measurement of and accountability for the quality of delivered services.

- Traditional indemnity health insurance is shrinking as a source of payment for health care, as is the fee-for-service care it financed, and indemnity insurers are either abandoning health insurance entirely, or are providing both indemnity insurance and managed care options, or are shifting to managed care entirely.

- Managed care organizations (MCOs), which combine both insurance and delivery functions, have become the most visible manifestation of change in the delivery system[1] (Luft and Greenlick, 1996).

---

[1]Managed care organizations include traditional group- and staff-model health maintenance organizations (HMOs), such as Kaiser-Permanente and Group Health

1

- A number of MCOs are now evolving into *integrated delivery systems*, which combine aspects of managed care with hospital-based delivery systems (Shortell et al., 1994).

- Simultaneously, the hospital is being displaced as the center of the health care system and the hospital sector is downsizing (both by reducing the number of beds and by closing hospitals), consolidating into multi-hospital chains, and evolving toward integrated delivery systems (Robinson, 1994; Stoeckle, 1995; Shortell et al., 1995).

- Physician practice is changing from traditional solo fee-for-service to single- and multi-specialty group practices that are contracting with managed care plans and, increasingly, are capitated, involve other risk-sharing arrangements, or involve physicians organizing health plans themselves.

Two primary concerns are driving the rate and direction of change. First, health care expenditures have imposed increasing burdens on federal and state governments, private employers, and individuals in recent years, stimulating a search for ways to control costs. Second, the concern that the quality of health care not be impaired by cost containment is encouraging a search for value received for the health care dollar spent.

In this overall context, medical technology is of substantial interest to many parties. The Office of Technology Assessment (OTA) defines *medical technology* as "the drugs, devices, and medical and surgical procedures used in medical care, and the organizational and supportive systems within which such care is provided" (Banta et al., 1981). This definition, which has been adopted by most analysts, embraces innovations in medicine—new drugs, biologics, medical devices, and procedures—as well as existing therapeutic and diagnostic capabilities.

Cooperative of Puget Sound, preferred provider organizations (PPOs), independent practice associations (IPAs), and network and mixed models; major health insurers that have converted, or are converting, wholly or in large part, from indemnity insurance to managed care, such as Prudential, Aetna, and CIGNA; and Blue Cross and Blue Shield Plans that are making a similar transition while usually remaining not-for-profit, although some notable cases (such as Wellpoint in California) are converting to for-profit status.

At least three reasons can be given for the interest in medical technology. First, it is believed by many to be a major driver of increased health expenditures (Weisbrod, 1991; Newhouse, 1993; Rettig, 1994; Cutler, 1995), and, thus, an object of cost containment. Second, medical technology is also regarded as a primary guarantor of quality in U.S. health care. Third, both elite and public opinions strongly support innovation in medicine as the hoped-for source of tomorrow's solutions to many of today's intractable medical problems, such as AIDS, cancer, and diabetes. These attitudes toward medical technology create great ambivalence among makers of both public and private health policy, who wish to control the likely increased costs of medical technology without sacrificing the benefits of innovation. This ambivalence has often complicated efforts, especially in the public sector, to establish effective institutions and processes for evaluating the benefits and costs of medical technology.

Against this background, evaluation of the clinical effectiveness and cost-effectiveness of medical technology is a matter of great concern to a diverse number of institutions—purchasers, insurers, managed care organizations, hospitals, physicians, other health care personnel, and patients. *Technology assessment* (TA), the term most often applied to such evaluation, was defined by an Institute of Medicine (IOM) report (IOM—Mosteller, 1985, p. 2) as "any process of examining and reporting properties of a medical technology used in health care, such as safety, efficacy, feasibility, and indications for use, cost, and cost-effectiveness, as well as social, economic, and ethical consequences, whether intended or unintended." Although not included in the definition, the distinction between *efficacy*, or "what a method [technology] can accomplish in expert hands when correctly applied to an appropriate patient" and *effectiveness*, or a technology's "performance in more general routine applications" is discussed in the report.

Several reports have assessed the status of TA in medicine over time. In 1985, the Institute of Medicine published *Assessing Medical Technologies* (IOM—Mosteller, 1985), which surveyed the field of TA and included profiles of 20 organizations that conducted TA programs. These programs fell into the following categories: professional medical societies, the hospital sector, third-party insurers, health maintenance organizations, therapeutic products firms and industries (pharmaceutical, biotechnology, medical device), TA consulting and research organizations, and federal government agencies (biomedical research, health services research, technology assessment, information resources, health policy analysis, and reimbursement-related policy analysis).

In 1988, the IOM published the *Medical Technology Assessment Directory* (IOM—Goodman, 1988), which greatly expanded the number of TA organizational profiles and added information on specific medical technologies, TA information resources, and TA organizational resources. The *Directory* used the same organizational categories as the 1985 report, but added federal government regulatory and payment agencies and many international organizations.

A 1994 Office of Technology Assessment report, *Identifying Health Technologies That Work: Searching for Evidence*, is the most recent review. With 954 references, it is undoubtedly the most extensive survey of the literature. Although the report emphasizes federal government agencies involved in TA and clinical practice guidelines development, it observes that the private-sector market for technology assessment was "small but explosive," thus raising the broad question that motivated this study.

THE CHANGING CONTEXT OF TECHNOLOGY ASSESSMENT

The historical experience with technology assessment in the United States has been mixed. In brief, it has involved the aspiration for a federal government leadership role in TA, the unrealized fulfillment of that aspiration, and the emergence of a strong private-sector TA capability in recent years. The aspiration of many advocates has long been to establish a federal government leadership role in TA, the high point of which came in the mid-1970s. Beginning with the establishment in 1974 of a Health Program within the Office of Technology Assessment of the U.S. Congress, these initiatives also included the adoption of the Medical Device Amendments of 1976, which expanded the role of the Food and Drug Administration (FDA), the creation in 1977 of the Office of Medical Applications of Research within the National Institutes of Health, and the creation of the National Center for Health Care Technology (NCHCT) in 1978.

High hopes for federal government TA leadership were embodied in NCHCT, which existed within the U.S. Public Health Service from

1978 through 1982 (Perry, 1982; Blumenthal, 1983; Rettig, 1991). These hopes were abruptly dashed in 1981, however, after the inauguration of President Ronald Reagan. Although Congress reauthorized NCHCT that year, it failed to appropriate any funds for its continued operation. When the agency ceased to function in 1982, a national, nongovernmental, public-private entity was advocated (Bunker et al., 1982b; IOM—Barondess, 1983). In response, after Congress authorized it in 1984 and 1985, the Council on Health Care Technology was established within the Institute of Medicine (NIH). This body, which existed from 1985 to 1989, did not become an effective assessment agency, and when Congress withdrew the statutory authority for its public funding in 1989, the IOM discontinued it.

The period that began in the mid-1970s effectively ended in 1989 with the termination of the IOM's Council, the creation of the Agency for Health Care Policy and Research (AHCPR), and the assumption by AHCPR of responsibility for the Office of Health Technology Assessment (OHTA).

One aspect of the federal government's role in TA has been the efforts over an extended period by the Health Care Financing Administration (HCFA) to strengthen the evaluative rigor of its coverage-decision processes. HCFA's source of advice within the federal government historically has been the Public Health Service (PHS). This Medicare-delegated PHS function has been exercised by NCHCT (1978–1982) and, from 1982 to the present, by the Office of Health Technology Assessment. One notable feature of the HCFA experience was the issuance in 1989 of a proposed rule that would add a cost-effectiveness element to the analyses supporting coverage and payment decisions (54 FR 4302, January 30, 1989). A final rule has been described as "imminent" for several years.

Given the prominence of HCFA as a purchaser of health care services through Medicare and Medicaid, and given the contribution those programs make to federal and state government budgets, it might be assumed that HCFA-as-purchaser would have developed a strong TA capability. In economic terms, the more fully informed about market transactions all parties are, the more efficiently markets perform. TA, at bottom, is one way of increasing the information available to purchasers of care about what works in medicine. There are also beneficial spillovers to private-sector health care from government-generated information about effectiveness: Such information is in the public domain and thus is available for the use of all other purchasers.

Historically, however, strong political opposition has existed, and will continue to exist, to the exercise by the federal government of a strong TA role. In the opinion of the therapeutic products industries, especially the medical devices industry (HIMA, 1995a–c), government TA is biased against innovation and in favor of cost containment. Thus, the substantial market power of HCFA that is exercised through Medicare is feared, and a stronger Medicare TA capability is steadfastly resisted. Critics of a strong HCFA TA effort, including the firms and trade associations of the therapeutic products industries, display relatively little concern about theoretical improvements in market efficiency as a result of better information when such information may challenge their economic self-interest.

The federal government picture would not be complete without mention of the Department of Veterans Affairs (DVA) and the Department of Defense (DoD). In many respects, DVA has been shielded from the intensity of the budgetary pressures that are acting on almost all other government agencies. Its hospital system has not been subjected to the same forces that are at work in the private sector. Consequently, it is only now beginning to develop a TA system. CHAMPUS (Civilian Health and Medical Program of the Uniformed Services), the DoD's insurance program for the dependents of military personnel, has taken a different route, contracting recently with the Blue Cross Blue Shield Association for a TA program rather than creating its own.

Although the federal government, from the mid-1970s to the present, has raised consciousness about TA and has enabled researchers to work out the analytical methods of TA, a strong federal government leadership role in TA has not emerged. Federal government agencies have failed politically to develop a constituency for TA and have actually developed some residual political enemies.

Neither the economic rationale for TA, which stems from HCFA's role as a major puchaser of health care services, nor the argument that federal government TA generates a spillover contribution to the entire U.S. health care system has been politically persuasive. Until political support for TA conducted or supported by the federal government has been established, the federal government's leadership role will remain unrealized.

This history of political failure notwithstanding, the idea of a national TA entity continues to receive support. Had the federal health care reform legislation proposed in 1993 become law, a strong federal government TA organization might have been established. In fact, the Physician Payment Review Commission (PPRC) recommended in early 1994 that a single national organization be established to conduct assessments supporting coverage decisions about new medical technologies (PPRC, 1994). However, in the wake of the collapse of reform legislation in 1994 and the election in November of that year of a Republican-controlled Congress, political support for such an approach to TA has all but vanished. A two-decade history of failed efforts to establish a strong federal or national TA organization reflects the ambivalence with which TA is regarded at the national level, as well as the limited political feasibility of such proposals.

THE RESEARCH QUESTIONS

In *Identifying Health Technologies That Work,* OTA (1994) argued that "the explosive growth in the private-sector market for the assessment of specific medical technologies" is one of the most significant developments in TA. Although some payers and providers have had long-standing TA programs, the report noted, "what is new is the degree to which technology assessments are becoming a standard ingredient in private-sector decisionmaking" (p. 9). And while the assessment of specific technologies by the federal government has been stable, "the private market in health technology assessments has become a full-fledged economic activity in its own right."

It is this observation about private-sector TA that provides the primary impetus for this report. By focusing on private-sector TA, we raise the following five questions for this study:

- What is the demand for TA?
- Who performs TA?

- What characterizes the content of TA?

- How are the results of TA used?

- What is the TA role of the federal government in light of these developments?

1. What Is the Demand for Technology Assessment?

The 1994 OTA report that argued that the private-sector market for technology assessment was "small but explosive" provided little evidence to support that claim. In this study, we examine whether the private-sector demand for TA is increasing—either steadily or explosively. If it is, how, and for what reasons? What organizations are driving change and why? What are the implications of changed demand on the conduct of TAs, especially on their rigor? Is increased demand resulting in TA being incorporated into decisionmaking policies and procedures of health care organizations? Is TA being integrated with other evaluative activities such as guidelines development? What expectations about the demand for TA are reasonable in the immediate future? These issues are considered in this chapter.

2. Who Performs Technology Assessment?

Private-sector organizations have been engaged in TA for some time, as two Institute of Medicine documents (1985, 1988) make clear. However, the assertion by OTA about the rapid growth of private-sector TA casts the discussion in a new light. In this study, we describe a number of the private health care organizations that are engaged in conducting technology assessment. What do they do? For whom? At what level of effort by professional staff and in volume of output? Are their TAs available freely or at nominal cost to the public, available only to organization members, or available on a subscription basis? What coordination, if any, exists among these TA performers? Some answers to these questions are provided in Chapter Two.

In our judgment, the data provided by the organizations interviewed for the study support the conclusion that substantial private-sector activity in TA is occurring, and from them we can formulate hypotheses that could be tested in a more comprehensive examination of private-sector activity in TA and the management of medical technology.

3. What Characterizes the Content of Technology Assessment?

The concern for performers of TA leads naturally to an examination of the content of assessments—the analytical and methodological strategies that characterize TA today. How is TA defined operationally? Are TAs typically evidence-based or based on expert consensus? What is the scope of TA and how has it changed in the decade? How are priorities for assessments established? What analytical techniques, including cost-effectiveness analysis, are used? What are the products (reports, papers, guidelines, coverage policies) of TAs? What TA resources are used? How is TA related to other evaluative activities, such as appropriateness, effectiveness, and outcomes research, and, especially, to the development of clinical practice guidelines? Chapter Three addresses these questions.

4. What Use Is Made of Technology Assessment Results?

The TA literature emphasizes how to perform assessments, rather than how these assessments can or should be used. Chapter Four discusses who uses TAs and for what purposes. What existing policies and procedures pertain to the implementation of TAs? Who is involved in decisions about the use of TAs? How are TAs evaluated for their clinical and financial utility?

5. What Is the Role of the Government?

Both the public and private sectors of health care have a large stake in the effective conduct and use of technology assessments. Given that a federal government TA leadership role has not emerged and that extensive private-sector TA has increasingly filled that gap, appropriate roles of each sector become an issue: What are the opportunities for constructive TA-related relationships—cooperation, collaboration, coordination, contracting, technical assistance—between the federal government and the private, nongovernmental health sector? A discussion of these issues concludes the study and is found in Chapter Five.

RESEARCH METHODS

Scope

The scope of this study, initially very broad, was narrowed in the early stages to a focus on managed care, because of time and resource constraints and because managed care constitutes the most significant change in the financing and delivery of health care. Managed care organizations have strong incentives to hold down the costs of care, and one way to do so is to avoid providing unnecessary, inappropriate, or inadequately tested medical technologies and procedures. Managed care has had, and is having, a strong but *indirect* effect on shrinking the demand for medical technology by reducing both hospital bed capacity and the demand for physician specialists. Presumably, it is also having a *direct* effect by dampening the incentives to purchase medical technology. This study was guided, therefore, by the assumption that managed care has strong incentives to evaluate medical technology for both clinical effectiveness and cost-effectiveness, incentives stronger than those in the other sectors.

However, a comprehensive analysis of private-sector TA would consider three other sectors of the health care system in addition to the insurance/managed care sector: hospitals, professional medical societies, and firms in the therapeutic products industries (pharmaceutical, biotechnology, and medical device). These four sectors differ in the incentives they have to develop, promote, and use medical technology and thus in their reasons for supporting or using technology assessments.

This study gives only limited consideration to the hospital sector and to professional medical societies, and none to the therapeutic products industries. The hospital sector has a complicated orientation toward technology and TA. Although medical technology may be viewed, in general, as a factor driving increasing costs of health care, or as underevaluated relative to patient outcomes, hospitals have confronted conflicting pressures regarding the use of medical technology. Medical technology has often been seen as a way to attract and retain physicians, to attract patients, and for a given hospital in a local market to differentiate itself from its competitors (Teplensky et al., 1995). Mainly, however, hospitals have seen technology as a revenue source.

As managed care has increased in importance, a conceptual shift has occurred, and former revenue centers have now come to be seen as cost centers. This shift in perception creates greater incentives in the hospital sector to engage in and use TA. Although its interest in TA has increased somewhat, the hospital sector historically has not been a strong source of demand for TA (Greer, 1985, 1987; Anderson and Steinberg, 1994; Teplensky et al., 1995). In the hospital sector, this study considers only the American Hospital Association (AHA) and the University HealthSystem Consortium (UHC). The former is the nation's largest hospital trade association. The latter, whose membership consists mainly of major academic teaching hospitals, has a strong TA program. A more detailed examination of the changing role of TA in the hospital sector is warranted.

Physician specialty societies accounted for a number of the entries in the 1988 Institute of Medicine *Directory*. In this study, we have included only the American Medical Association (AMA) and the American College of Physicians (ACP), on the assumption that, in 1995, physician specialty societies were more likely to be engaged in developing clinical practice guidelines than in performing technology assessments. Practice guidelines, after all, constitute one domain in which the medical profession has a high likelihood of asserting, or reasserting, professional control over its own activities. Indeed, both the AMA's Diagnostic and Therapeutic Technology Assessment Program and the ACP's Clinical Efficacy Assessment Program could be regarded as guidelines-development programs rather than as TA programs.

The firms and associations in the therapeutic products industries (pharmaceutical, biotechnology, and medical device) respond differently to TA as a function of their respective industry structures, their products, and the relative importance they attach to Food and Drug Administration regulatory issues and to insurance and managed care coverage and reimbursement decisions. The pharmaceutical industry has a more-or-less settled, even if fractious, relationship with FDA and is engaged actively in responding to the implications of pricing and marketing its products for a managed care world. In particular, it has stimulated the development of the field of "pharmacoeconomics," or the economics of the drug industry, and the inclusion of cost-effectiveness and quality-of-life analyses (i.e., the measurement of functional status, health status, and general well-being, using patient-reported data) in clinical trials. These activities help in making product-development decisions, in marketing products relative to competitors', and in preparing firms for a time when such tools are more widely used by public and private purchasers of care.

The biotechnology firms are preoccupied mainly with the FDA's drug and biologics review-and-approval process, and, therefore, with demonstrating the safety and efficacy of their products by randomized, controlled clinical trials.

The medical device industry stands in a somewhat different position from that of the pharmaceutical industry. Actively concerned with FDA reform of device evaluation, issues of product liability, and how to pay for clinical trials, the device industry focuses its concern on the "TA issues" of coverage and reimbursement, mainly by Medicare, less so by decentralized managed care organizations (HIMA, 1995c). Although we give no attention in this report to the firms in these industries, a thorough treatment of their views of TA is warranted.

Data Collection

We collected data by several methods: site visits; semi-structured interviews, both face-to-face and by telephone; attendance at meetings; document review; and follow-up on referrals to others.

We established contacts with the Blue Cross Blue Shield Association (BCBSA) and ECRI[2] early in the study, since, in 1995, both had been involved in TA for a long time. These contacts resulted in visits to both organizations. The initial visit to BCBSA involved a 1-hour interview with the principals of the Technology Evaluation Center (TEC), which laid the basis for later interviews with the medical

---

[2]ECRI was once known as the Emergency Care Research Institute, but has long since given up that name for the acronym.

directors of Blue Shield of California, Blue Cross Blue Shield of Illinois, Blue Cross Blue Shield of Minnesota, and Blue Cross Blue Shield of Oregon. Later, the author attended the two-day June 1995 meeting of TEC's Medical Advisory Panel as an observer. With ECRI, the visit resulted in a 6-hour detailed discussion with the directors of that organization's TA effort.

Site visits were made to Philadelphia (ECRI, the American College of Physicians, University of Pennsylvania, Jefferson University); Chicago (BCBSA, the American Medical Association, the American Hospital Association, the University HealthSystem Consortium, and Blue Cross Blue Shield of Illinois); San Francisco (Blue Shield of California, Kaiser-Permanente of Northern California); Minneapolis– St. Paul (University of Minnesota, HealthPartners, Institute for Clinical Systems Integration, Blue Cross Blue Shield of Minnesota, Allina Health System, Minnesota Business Health Care Action Group, and Medical Alley[3]); Seattle (Group Health Cooperative of Puget Sound); Portland (Blue Cross Blue Shield of Oregon); Los Angeles (Kaiser-Permanente of Southern California); and Hartford (Aetna).

All site visits involved face-to-face interviews of at least 1 hour; many resulted in extended discussions, including ECRI and the University HealthSystem Consortium; and several included multiple inter-views—for example, Group Health Cooperative of Puget Sound. The variation in length reflected the complexity of the organization's TA efforts. Some visits were preceded by telephone interviews, and some led to follow-up discussions on the telephone or in person when key individuals in these organizations visited Washington, DC. Toward the end of the project, a number of interviews were con-ducted by telephone and typically lasted 45 minutes to 1 hour. In all, 46 interviews were conducted with 56 individuals in 29 different or-ganizations. The brief snapshots of performers presented in Chapter Two were sent to the individual organizations for a review of accu-racy. (The list of the individuals interviewed and their organizational affiliations appears in the appendix to this chapter.)

The author also attended a meeting of the American College of Physicians' Subcommittee on Clinical Efficacy Assessment and a

---

[3]Medical Alley is an association of Minnesota health care organizations, most of which are medical device companies.

meeting of the Medical Policy Committee on Quality and Technology of Blue Shield of California.

SOURCES OF INCREASED DEMAND FOR TA

Whether the growth in private-sector TA has been "explosive" or not is less important than the basic questions that the OTA report (1994) raises. Has the demand for TA increased in recent years? If so, what accounts for this increased demand? What are the effects of this increased demand? This section considers these questions.

Demand, for purposes of this analysis, consists of a perceived need and willingness to pay for that need to be met. The response of suppliers who are potentially able to fulfill that need will vary as the strength of demand varies. The expression of demand is necessary to elicit a response from suppliers. For TA, *demand* is usually expressed in relation to other evaluative activities, which may include outcomes research, appropriateness research, clinical practice guidelines, and report cards. Although TA may sometimes be requested alone, more often it is nested in a set of complementary evaluative efforts that are usually linked to managing the utilization of health services and to quality assurance or improvement of those services.

Currently, the priority of the health care marketplace, especially in the private sector, is to control the costs of health care. At the same time, however, many purchasers and providers are also giving substantial attention to quality of care, or to the value of the health care received for the resources expended. This dual concern for costs and value provides the basis for the increased demand for TA (IOM–Field and Shapiro, 1993, pp. 223–227).

In this cost-value context, there are two main sources of increased private-sector demand for TA. The first is the major corporate purchasers of health care, especially self-insured corporations, which have pressed for both cost containment and performance evaluation (Darling, 1991). The second main source of demand is major health care insurers and managed care plans, which have found TA useful in responding to the changing health care marketplace—to health care purchasers, to increasingly severe economic constraints, and, prospectively, to patients.

In general, large corporations, especially the self-insured, have become a major force in the health care sector for encouraging the containment of costs and raising the issue of value received for funds spent (Freudenheim, 1995). A 1993 Institute of Medicine report (IOM–Field and Shapiro, p. 216) found that the evidence that employer cost-containment strategies had limited the growth of health care costs was "at best, quite modest, although certain techniques appear to have reduced some unnecessary or inappropriate spending and some have shifted a portion of the cost burden from employers to employees" (p. 216). More-recent analyses document a much more aggressive and effective role by health care purchasers in containing costs (Robinson, 1995).

Patricelli (1994) has argued that self-insured employers have driven much of the innovation in the financing and delivery of care:

> Any practitioner of managed care knows that large, self-insured employers have driven the development of most of the advances in managed care technology in this country. The reasons are simple. These employers have sophisticated staffs who can challenge and work with managed care vendors, and they do so because they are self-insured and get the economic benefit of any savings they generate. . . . Moreover, innovations including claims data analysis, utilization review, high-cost case management, point-of-service options, flex plans, carve-out specialty managed care plans, centers of excellence, and quality measurement in health care all have originated from vendor interactions with self-insured employers.

Self-insured employers, for example, have been instrumental in the development of the National Committee on Quality Assurance (NCQA), the primary accrediting body for health maintenance organizations (O'Kane, personal communication, 1995; Darling, 1995; Iglehart, 1996). In particular, performance evaluation, as reflected in the Health Plan and Employer Data and Information Set (HEDIS) report cards, is a clear instance of purchaser-driven demand for information about quality (Allen et al., 1994; Roper, 1995). As another example, in mid-1995, the *New York Times* reported that, at a Jackson Hole, Wyoming, meeting, representatives of some of the largest employers and purchasers of health insurance had agreed to pursue a fundamental shift in emphasis in the nation's managed care systems: "They want the primary focus to be placed on measuring the quality of care now that costs have begun to be controlled" (Noble, 1995).

Perhaps the most significant development in the private demand for TA has been the addition by NCQA of a TA-utilization-management requirement to its accreditation standards (NCQA, 1995). Requirement U.M. 7.0, which became effective on April 1, 1995, states that

> the managed care organization has policies and procedures in place to evaluate the appropriate use of new medical technologies, or new applications of established technologies, including medical procedures, drugs, and devices.

Although sparing of details about precise organization of the TA effort, this requirement specifies that "appropriate professionals" be involved in the development of evaluation criteria, that such criteria include "review of information from appropriate government regulatory bodies and published scientific evidence," and that these criteria be used "effectively" to assess both new technologies and new applications of existing technologies. Therefore, to the extent that managed care plans seek NCQA accreditation, and major corporate purchasers are encouraging them to do so, this requirement is a strong indication of private-sector demand for TA.

Regional groups of purchasers also have exerted strong influence on providers in local health care markets. Prominent among these are the Washington Business Group on Health, the Midwest Business Group on Health, the Pacific Business Group on Health, and the Minnesota Business Health Care Action Group (BHCAG).

The BHCAG, whose members include the major self-insured corporations in Minnesota, has taken an active role in health care organization and delivery. In 1992, it issued a Request for Proposals to the major provider organizations in the state, requiring that acceptable responses provide for clinical practice guidelines and technology assessment. The winning proposal from HealthPartners resulted in the establishment of the Institute for Clinical Systems Integration (ICSI). ICSI is a separate organization that develops guidelines and conducts TAs for use in coverage and reimbursement by HealthPartners and some 20 other participating health plans. (ICSI is described in greater detail in Chapter Two.)

The second source of increased demand for TA comes from the insurance and managed care organizations themselves. These organizations are responding primarily to the demands placed on them by major purchasers of care, but they are also acting in accordance with their own strategic appraisals of both the immediate and longer-term requirements for survival in the competitive health care market. Although MCOs have cost containment as a primary objective, they are also concerned with quality issues. These dual concerns manifest themselves in the establishment of a set of evaluative activities, among which TA is an element. MCOs are a source of demand for TA in health care, making possible, for example, the growth of the TA subscription services of the Blue Cross Blue Shield Association and ECRI.

REFERENCES

Allen, H.M., Darling, H., McNeill, D.N., Bastien, F., 1994. "The employee health care value survey: round one," *Health Affairs*, Vol. 13, No. 4 (Fall), pp. 25–41.

Anderson, G.F., and Steinberg, E.P., 1994. "Role of the hospital in the acquisition of technology," in Gelijns, A.C., and Dawkins, H.V., eds., 1994. *Adopting New Medical Technology: Medical Innovation at the Crossroads, Vol. IV*, Washington, DC, National Academy Press, pp. 61–70.

Banta, H.D., Behney, C.J., and Sisk, J.S., 1981. *Toward Rational Technology in Medicine*, New York, Springer Publishing Company.

Blumenthal, D., 1983. "Federal policy toward health care technology: the case of the National Center," *Milbank Memorial Fund Quarterly/Health and Society*, Vol. 61, pp. 584–613.

Brook, R.H., Park, R.E., Chassin, M.R., Solomon, D.H., Keesey, J., Kosecoff, J., 1990. "Predicting the appropriate use of carotid endarterectomy, upper gastrointestinal endoscopy, and coronary angiography," *New England Journal of Medicine*, Vol. 323, pp. 1173–1177.

Bunker, J.P., Fowles, J., Schaffarzick, R., 1982a. "Evaluation of medical technology strategies: effects of coverage and reimbursement," *New England Journal of Medicine*, Vol. 306, pp. 620–624.

Bunker, J.P., Fowles, J., Schaffarzick, R., 1982b. "Evaluation of medical technology strategies: proposal for an institute of health care evaluation," *New England Journal of Medicine*, Vol. 306, pp. 687–692.

Cutler, D.M., 1995. "Technology, health costs, and the NIH," paper prepared for the National Institutes of Health Economics Roundtable on Biomedical Research, Bethesda, MD.

Darling, H., 1991. "Employers and managed care: what are the early returns?" *Health Affairs*, Vol. 10, No. 4 (Winter), pp. 147–160.

Darling, H., 1995. "Market reform: large corporations lead the way," *Health Affairs*, Vol. 14, No. 1 (Spring), pp. 122–124.

Freudenheim, M., 1995. "10 companies join in effort to lower bids by HMOs," *New York Times*, May 23.

Fryback, D.G., ed., 1995. *Introduction to Technology Assessment for Radiologists: Vision Beyond Tomorrow*, Vols. 1 and 2, Milwaukee, WI, GE Medical Systems–Association of University Radiologists Radiology Research Academic Fellowship (GERRAF) Program.

Greer, A.L., 1985. "Adoption of medical technology: the hospital's three decision systems," *International Journal of Technology Assessment in Health Care*, Vol. 1, No. 5, pp. 669–680.

Greer, A.L., 1987. "Rationing medical technology: hospital decision-making in the United States," *International Journal of Technology Assessment in Health Care*, Vol. 3, No. 2, pp. 199–222.

Health Industry Manufacturers Association (HIMA), 1995a. *Report on Public Policy Reform and the U.S. Health Care Technology Industry. Part I: Reforms at the Food and Drug Administration*, Washington, DC, February 9.

Health Industry Manufacturers Association (HIMA), 1995b. *Report on Public Policy Reform and the U.S. Health Care Technology Industry. Part II: Reforming Product Liability Laws*, Washington, DC, March 2.

Health Industry Manufacturers Association (HIMA), 1995c. *Report on Public Policy Reform and the U.S. Health Care Technology Industry. Part III: Strengthening the Climate for Health Care Financing and Delivery*, Washington, DC, May 5.

Iglehart, J.K., 1996. "The National Committee for Quality Assurance," *New England Journal of Medicine*, Vol. 335, No. 13, pp. 995–999.

Institute of Medicine (IOM–Barondess, J., ed.), 1983. *A Consortium for Assessing Medical Technology*, Washington, DC, National Academy Press.

Institute of Medicine (IOM—Field, M.J., and Shapiro, H.T., eds.), 1993. *Employment and Health Benefits: A Connection at Risk*, Washington, DC, National Academy Press.

Institute of Medicine (IOM—Goodman, C., ed.), 1988. *Medical Technology Assessment Directory*, Washington, DC, National Academy Press.

Institute of Medicine (IOM—Mosteller, F., ed.), 1985. *Assessing Medical Technologies*, Washington, DC, National Academy Press.

Luft, H.S., and Greenlick, H.R., 1996. "The role and contributions of managed care: 1. The contribution of group- and staff-model HMOs to American medicine," *Milbank Quarterly*, Vol. 74, No. 4, pp. 445–468.

Mendelson, D.N., Abramson, R.G., and Rubin, R.J., 1995. "State involvement in medical technology assessment," *Health Affairs*, Vol. 14, No. 2 (Summer), pp. 83–98.

National Committee for Quality Assurance (NCQA), 1995. *Standards for Accreditation*, Washington, DC.

Newhouse, J.P., 1993. "An iconoclastic view of health cost containment," *Health Affairs*, Vol. 12 (Suppl.), pp. 152–171.

Noble, H.B., 1995. "Quality is focus for health plans," *New York Times*, July 3.

Office of Technology Assessment (OTA), U.S. Congress, 1994. *Identifying Health Technologies That Work: Searching for Evidence*, Washington, DC, U.S. Government Printing Office.

Patricelli, R.E., 1994. "Why do we need health alliances?" *Health Affairs*, Vol. 13, No. 1 (Spring), pp. 239–242.

Perry, S., 1982. "The brief life of the National Center for Health Care Technology," *New England Journal of Medicine*, Vol. 307, pp. 1095–1100.

Physician Payment Review Commission (PPRC), 1994. *Annual Report to Congress, 1994*, Washington, DC, pp. 219–236.

Rettig, R.A., 1991. "Technology assessment: an update," *Investigative Radiology*, Vol. 26, pp. 165–173.

Rettig, R.A., 1994. "Medical innovation duels cost containment," *Health Affairs*, Vol. 13, No. 3 (Summer), pp. 7–27.

Robinson, J.C., 1994. "The changing boundaries of the American hospital," *Milbank Quarterly*, Vol. 72, No. 2, pp. 259–275.

Robinson, J.C., 1995. "Health care purchasing and market changes in California," *Health Affairs*, Vol. 14, No. 4 (Winter), pp. 117–130.

Roper, W.L., 1995. "Quality assurance in the competitive marketplace," *Health Affairs*, Vol. 14, No. 1 (Spring), pp. 120–121.

Shortell, S.M., Gillies, R.R., and Anderson, D.A., 1994. "The new world of managed care: creating organized delivery systems," *Health Affairs*, Vol. 13, No. 5, Winter, pp. 46–64.

Shortell, S.M., Gillies, R.R., and Devers, K.J., 1995. "Reinventing the American hospital," *Milbank Quarterly*, Vol. 73, No. 2, pp. 131–160.

Stoeckle, J.D., 1995. "The citadel cannot hold: technologies go outside the hospital, patients and doctors too," *Milbank Quarterly*, Vol. 73, No. 1, pp. 3–17.

Teplensky, J.D., Pauly, M.V., Kimberly, J.R., Hillman, A.L., and Schwartz, J.S., 1995. "Hospital adoption of medical technology: an empirical test of alternative models," *HSR: Health Services Research*, Vol. 30, No. 3 (August), pp. 437–465.

Weisbrod, B.A., 1991. "The health care quadrilemma: an essay on technological change, insurance, quality of care, and cost containment," *Journal of Economic Literature*, Vol. 29, pp. 523–552.

Wennberg, J.E., Freeman, J.L., and Culp, W.J., 1987. "Are hospital services rationed in New Haven or over-utilized in Boston?" *The Lancet*, Vol. 1 (May 23), pp. 1185–1188.

Wennberg, J.E., and Gittlesohn, A., 1982. "Variations in medical care among small areas," *Scientific American*, Vol. 246, pp. 120–134.

Wennberg, J.E., and Gittlesohn, A., 1983. "Small area variations in health care delivery," *Science*, Vol. 142, pp. 1102–1108.

Appendix:
INTERVIEWS FOR THE TA STATUS PROJECT

Third-party insurers and managed care organizations:

- Aetna: William T. McGiveney

- Allina: Gordon M. Sprenger, John H. Kleinman*

- Blue Cross Blue Shield Association: Susan Gleeson, Naomi Aronson, Ellen Pearson; the author also attended June 29, 1995, meeting of Medical Advisory Panel

- Blue Cross Blue Shield of Minnesota: Del Ohrt, Jack Alexander, Julie Carr

- Blue Cross Blue Shield of Illinois: Arnold L. Widen

- Blue Cross Blue Shield of Oregon: John Santa

- Blue Shield of California: Wade M. Aubry; the author also attended June 7, 1995, meeting of Medical Policy Committee on Quality and Technology

- CIGNA: Edward J. Smith,* Jadwiga Goclowski*

- Group Health Cooperative of Puget Sound, Seattle, Washington: Hugh Straley, Terri Calnan, Simeon Rubenstein, Michael E. Stuart,* Jeff K. Shornick, Timothy McAfee, Edward H. Wagner*

- Harvard Community Health Plan, Boston, Massachusetts: Melinda Karp*

- HAYES: Winifred S. Hays

- Health Partners, Minneapolis, Minnesota: George J. Isham

- The HMO Group, New Brunswick, N.J., and TEMINEX, Buffalo, New York: Daniel Wolfson,* John Reinhard*

- Institute for Clinical Systems Integration, Minneapolis, Minnesota: Gordon Mosser, James C. Smith

- Kaiser-Permanente Program: Ian Leverton*

---

*Telephone interview.

- Kaiser-Permanente Medical Group of Northern California: D. Blair Beebe,* Joseph Selby

- Kaiser-Permanente Medical Group of Southern California: Les Zendle, Robin Cisneros, David Eddy*

- Prudential: Arthur L. Levin,* William L. Roper*

- United HealthCare: Lee N. Newcomer,* Joseph A. Barry,* Sylvia Giebler Robinson*

Other organizations:

- American College of Physicians: Linda J. White; the author also attended May 31, 1995, meeting of Clinical Efficacy Assessment Subcommittee

- American Hospital Association: Suzanna Hoppszallern

- American Medical Association: Sona Kalousdian, Andrea Schneider

- ECRI: Jeffrey Lerner, Vivian Coates

- Medical Alley: Tom Meskan

- Minnesota Business Health Care Action Group: Steve Wetzel

- National Committee on Quality Assurance: Margaret E. O'Kane, Cary Sennet*

- Thomas Jefferson University: David Nash

- University Hospital Consortium (now University HealthSystem Consortium): David A. Burnett, Karl A Matuszewski, Jean Livingston, Richard A. Bankowtiz

- University of Pennsylvania: Alan Hillman, J. Sanford Schwarz

- Xerox: Helen Darling*

---

*Telephone interview.

Chapter Two

THE PERFORMERS OF TECHNOLOGY ASSESSMENT

The organizational reality of technology assessment in the mid-1990s is far more complex than what it was a decade earlier. It is highly decentralized, is becoming more so, and the performers are now located mainly in the private sector. In this chapter, we examine a number of private-sector organizations that perform TA. Although this report does not attempt to be comprehensive, it does characterize the nature and diversity of private-sector TA efforts.

Two Institute of Medicine reports in the mid-1980s provide some indication of the change that has taken place in the past decade. The 1985 report, *Assessing Medical Technologies* (IOM—Mosteller, 1985), listed 20 technology assessment programs. The 1988 *Medical Technology Assessment Directory* (IOM—Goodman, 1988), presented information on over 150 TA organizations and programs. The characteristics of the TA organizations and programs are worth noting. First, both documents, but especially the *Directory*, sought to include as many TA organizations or programs as possible, but did not group either by health care sector. Second, the lists were heavily weighted toward federal government agencies. Third, although the inclusion of the Blue Cross Blue Shield Association reflected its position as a TA pioneer in the 1970s and 1980s, the fact that it was the only insurer listed is evidence of the generally weak demand for TA among third-party payers in the mid-1980s. Fourth, medical societies, prominent on the IOM technology assessment lists, are engaged today as much, if not more so, in developing clinical practice guidelines.

To display the change that has occurred over time, we first present information on private TA performers that were clearly established a decade ago. We then discuss new (or newly visible) private-sector TA performers. The chapter concludes with summary observations about private-sector TA activity. We ask the following questions: What do these organizations do in technology assessment? For whom? At what level of effort by professional staff and in volume of output? Are their TAs available freely or at nominal cost to the public, available only to the organization's members, or available on a subscription basis? What coordination, if any, exists among these TA performers?

We considered preparing a tabular summary of data on these organizations, especially for full-time equivalent (FTE) personnel and number of assessments conducted each year. However, the diversity of organizations, programs, products, and staffing patterns was such that a tabular presentation would both be misleading and run the risk of being widely cited. We decided, instead, that narrative better served the purposes of the report.

PREVIOUSLY ESTABLISHED TA ORGANIZATIONS

Several organizations with TA roots in the 1970s have prospered in recent years. Several others that have conducted TA activities for a long time have undergone transitions that reflect external market changes, internal organizational changes, and strategic decisions about the priorities of the parent organizations. Our purpose was to describe these efforts, not to rank them by importance; therefore, we present previously established TA organizations in alphabetical order. In this section, we discuss the American College of Physicians, the American Hospital Association, the American Medical Association, the Blue Cross Blue Shield Association, Blue Shield of California, and ECRI.

American College of Physicians

The Clinical Efficacy Assessment Project (CEAP) of the American College of Physicians (ACP) began in 1981. CEAP evolved from ACP participation in the Medical Necessity Program of the Blue Cross Blue Shield Association (see below), from which it had received financial support for *Common Diagnostic Tests: Use and Interpretation* (Sox, 1987, 1990) and *Common Screening Tests* (Eddy,

1991). The CEAP program received a three-year grant from the Hartford Foundation in its initial years (1981–1984). It has been funded since from internal ACP funds and has relied heavily on its members voluntarily contributing their time to conduct its assessments.

CEAP assessments examine in detail a technology or procedure. Over time, the focus has expanded from evaluating the safety, efficacy, and effectiveness of diagnostic tests and medical technologies to assessing procedures and treatments used in clinical practice. The process involves a literature review and synthesis conducted by one or more college members, compilation of evidence tables (see Tables 3.2–3.6 in Chapter Three), and preparation of a manuscript by the analysts. The manuscript is subject to extensive review before it is published as a report authored by the analysts. A second product, generated by the CEAP committee, is a draft statement about the appropriate conclusions and recommendations to be drawn from the review-synthesis manuscript. This draft guideline is also subject to extensive review and, when approved by the College's Board of Regents, becomes the official position of the ACP.

Both the ACP-approved guideline and the analysts' background paper are submitted for publication to the *Annals of Internal Medicine*. Many assessments have been highly controversial, because they have intruded on the domains of various medical specialties, given that internal medicine intersects strongly with many specialty groups.

The ACP issues about 10 assessments each year, a figure that has been stable for most of the past decade. The challenge to the ACP is whether to continue CEAP as a modest, subsidized effort, whose products are free to interested parties, or to transform it in some way.

American Hospital Association

In 1982, the American Hospital Association (AHA) initiated the Hospital Technology Series program, which is built around a set of publications and educational programs. The purpose of this program was to help health-care managers keep abreast of both innovations in health technology and clinical hospital services and the implications that the innovations had for capital budgeting, staffing, training, maintenance, and the provision of clinical services. Financing came from internal AHA funds, from educational programs, and from publication revenues.

In the early 1990s, the AHA underwent a major reorganization when a new president moved the main office from Chicago to Washington, DC. Policy functions previously located in Chicago were moved to Washington because the organization was focusing its legislative energies on health care reform. Concurrently, all AHA products and services were reviewed. The Hospital Technology Series lost its internal AHA funding and the educational programs were cancelled, but the publications program was continued.

The Health Technology Series now includes *Hospital Technology Scanner* (a newsletter); reports containing evaluations of current and emerging management strategies, clinical practices, and medical technologies; and special reports that focus on current technology issues and trends. These publications are oriented mainly to hospital services—cardiology, clinical laboratory, diagnostic imaging, neurology, oncology, orthopedic services, rehabilitation, surgery, and to "big ticket" technologies such as information systems, lasers, lithotripters, magnetic resonance imaging (MRI), and positron emission tomography (PET).

Even this scaled-back effort reflects the continuing need of AHA members for technology assistance and the need of the organization to maintain a presence in this field. In 1995, the AHA signed an agreement with the University HealthSystem Consortium to market the latter's TA reports to AHA members.

American Medical Association

The American Medical Association (AMA) has long issued reports on the scientific bases of various clinical procedures. It initiated its Diagnostic and Therapeutic Technology Assessment (DATTA) program in 1982, publishing its first report in the *Journal of the American Medical Association* (*JAMA*) in 1983. The number of DATTA assessments has varied over time: it was approximately 10 per year from 1989 through 1991; then it fell in 1992 to five and remained at that level through 1994. This reduction in DATTA activity was due to a general retrenchment in AMA activities, precipitated by general financial pressures. This retrenchment was marked by a two-year va-cancy in the position of vice president for science and technology, the elimination of a long-standing drug-evaluation program, and the loss of many science and technology staff. Although the DATTA pro-gram was continued, its staff was reduced and the number of as-sessments scaled back.

The process by which DATTA assessments are conducted has changed over time. Previously, DATTA staff prepared questions about a technology and distributed them to a panel of about 20 physicians drawn from a pool of several thousand experts. The questionnaire was not accompanied by a literature review, although one had been prepared by the staff. The result was an opinion poll of a number of experts, which subjected the DATTA process to external criticism about the validity of expert consensus as a means of evaluating the science reported in the literature.

Under the new regime, questions are sent to a panel of expert physi-cians as before, but a literature review on which the questions are based is now sent to all panelists. The literature review, more sys-tematic and structured than before, is a staff product that is evalu-ated by 2–3 peer reviewers from different specialties and with different points of view. The review does not involve meta-analysis, a methodology for aggregating the results of clinical trials (see Chalmers, 1994). In addition, a simple analysis of the data pertaining to the technology accompanies the questionnaire. Panel respon-dents rate both the safety and effectiveness of each technology, using an ordinal scale from +2 to –2, corresponding to the following five dimensions: whether the technology is established, promising, in-vestigational, doubtful, or unacceptable. The size of the panels has been increased from about 20 individuals to about 50 at a minimum, often over 100, and sometimes as high as 250. Finally, if there are not enough experts in the pool, the DATTA program will go outside the pool to the needed specialists or will go to the appropriate specialty societies.

The DATTA program employs 2.5–3.0 FTE employees. Assessments today run 12–15 pages, compared with about 3 pages previously; many are published in *JAMA*; all are available on a subscription ser-vice basis. With a DATTA subscription, which costs $325 for one year and $485 for two years, come back copies of TAs; current assessments; current Tech Briefs (4–5-page documents describing a technology and the non–peer-reviewed results of a survey of a panel of experts); the DATTA newsletter, *Technology News;* and access to the DATTA clearinghouse. Of the 800–900 subscribers, 80 percent are medical doctors (M.D.s), most of whom are engaged in managed care and utilization review.

Blue Cross Blue Shield Association

Blue Cross Blue Shield Association began its TA effort in 1977 with its Medical Necessity program. Identifying obsolete medical procedures, the program aided member plans in determining whether to continue coverage of such procedures. The results of this program were made available publicly by periodic press releases. BCBSA then added a Technology Evaluation and Coverage program in the early 1980s to assist member plans in making coverage decisions about new medical technologies. However, the results of this program were available only to member plans.

BCBSA also actively supported the TA efforts of other organizations. Most notably, it financed *Common Diagnostic Tests: Use and Interpretation* (Sox, 1987, 1990) and *Common Screening Tests* (Eddy, 1991), both prepared and published by the American College of Physicians. It also provided financial support to the Institute of Medicine's Council on Health Care Technology from 1985 through 1989.

Over time, Medical Necessity and Technology Evaluation and Coverage efforts converged analytically. As they did, a business decision was made to offer the reports of both programs to the public—on a subscription basis—and not to seek a proprietary position on scientific information. In late 1993, BCBSA went public with an expanded technology assessment effort.

Three products are now available: at the low end, *Tecnologica*, a newsletter published 10 times a year, costs $400 per year and provides summary information on at least one assessment per issue; in the middle, a standard subscription of $13,500 buys all TA reports, which number approximately 40 per year, plus the newsletter; and at the high end, an additional customized package of services is available, including TA training of the subscriber's personnel and rights of observation at the BCBSA Medical Advisory Panel (MAP) meetings.

Concurrent with going public, BCBSA entered into a collaborative relationship with Kaiser-Permanente (KP), an arrangement regarded favorably by both parties. Both organizations are not-for-profit; both have invested substantial resources in quality-related efforts over time; BCBSA has a strong analytic staff; and KP has the largest HMO patient enrollment in the country. In this collaboration, both organizations share the services of Dr. David Eddy, a leading expert in TA; KP, with two representatives on the MAP, has access to the deliberations of the panel; and KP physicians are used in reviewing draft TAs, giving the final products a clinical reality test. At the same time that these changes were occurring, the MAP was changed to reduce the representation of Blue Cross members, add the two KP representatives, and appoint several unaffiliated national experts on TA and clinical research. Today, unaffiliated members constitute a majority of the MAP.

The BCBSA TA program had grown to about 20 assessments a year by the time the 1993 change occurred. From 1993 to 1994, however, the capacity and output doubled, and about 40 reports are now being produced each year. These reports are prepared by a full-time staff of approximately 10 Ph.D. and M.D. professionals, augmented by consultants as needed. Draft reports are reviewed by the MAP, which meets for four one-day meetings each year. The MAP considers the specific technologies on which staff have prepared reports, and discusses and votes on a staff recommendation that a given technology "does meet" or "does not meet" the BCBSA technology evaluation criteria (presented in Table 2.1). These reports are advisory to member plans and subscribers, an input to decisionmaking, usually for coverage decisions. BCBSA represents its work strictly as TAs, not as clinical practice guidelines.

Blue Shield of California

Among the individual plans of BCBSA, Blue Shield of California (BSC) stands out as having a long-established, well-developed TA program. The program, which is administered under the aegis of the Blue Shield Medical Director, revolves around the Medical Policy

Table 2.1

Blue Cross Blue Shield Association's Technology Evaluation Criteria

1. **The technology must have final approval from the appropriate government regulatory bodies.**

    - This criterion applies to drugs, biological products, devices and diagnostics.
    - A drug or biological product must have final approval from the Food and Drug Administration.
    - A device must have final approval from the Food and Drug Administration for those specific indications and methods of use that Blue Cross Blue Shield is evaluating.
    - Any approval that is granted as an interim step in the Food and Drug Administration regulatory process is not sufficient.

2. **The scientific evidence must permit conclusions concerning the effect of the technology on health outcomes.**

    - The evidence should consist of well-designed and well-conducted investigations published in peer-reviewed journals. The quality of the body of studies and the consistency of the results are considered in evaluating the evidence.
    - The evidence should demonstrate that the technology can measure or alter the physiological changes related to a disease, injury, illness, or condition. In addition, there should be evidence or a convincing argument based on established medical facts that such measurement or alteration affects health outcomes.
    - Opinions and evaluations by national medical associations, consensus panels, or other technology evaluation bodies are evaluated according to the scientific quality of the supporting evidence and rationale.

3. **The technology must improve the net health outcome.**

    - The technology's beneficial effects on health outcomes should outweigh any harmful effects on health outcomes.

4. **The technology must be as beneficial as any established alternative.**

    - The technology should improve the net health outcome as much as, or more than, established alternatives.

5. **The improvement must be attainable outside the investigational settings.**

    - When used under the usual conditions of medical practice, the technology should be reasonably expected to satisfy TEC Criteria #3 and #4.

SOURCE: Blue Cross Blue Shield Association, Chicago, Illinois. Reprinted by permission from the Blue Cross and Blue Shield Association.

Committee on Quality and Technology, a committee of the BSC Board of Directors. Most of the 18–20 committee members are BSC board members, but some non–board members are added for their expertise. Of the committee members, roughly two-thirds are M.D.s, one is an ethicist, and one is a lawyer.

The Medical Policy Committee meets three times each year. At each meeting it considers a half dozen or so "medical policy topics": new procedures or technologies for which a Blue Shield policy does not exist, or new indications for existing technologies for which a review and modification of a current policy are required. At the March 1995 meeting, for example, the agenda items were laser uterine nerve ablation (LUNA); stereotactic radiosurgery for multiple brain metastases and gliomas; positron emission tomography for oncology indications; sleep apnea testing; sleep apnea surgeries; prolotherapy; and obsolete medical policies. The agenda for the June 1995 meeting included cryosurgery of liver tumors; arthroscopy and arthroscopic surgery of the hip; stereotactic pallidotomy for Parkinson's disease; external insulin pump therapy; and intravenous immunoglobulin (IVIG) indications. The October 1995 agenda included stereotactic pallidotomy for Parkinson's disease (which had been discussed and tabled in June 1995); PET for oncology and cardiology indications (oncology indications were discussed and tabled in March, pending a BCBSA technology assessment; the BCBSA TA added cardiology indications); lung volume reduction surgery (LVRS); meniscal allograft transplantation; clinical indications for the use of plasmapheresis; and hyperbaric oxygen therapy.

For each of the medical technologies selected for consideration at any given meeting, the BSC process involves a staff-generated literature review. This review becomes the basis for a policy recommendation by the Medical Director to the Medical Policy Committee, accompanied by supporting documentation. The committee receives two notebooks before each meeting. The first notebook contains the staff analyses of the medical technologies or procedures under consideration. These analyses address the specific issue coming before the committee, relevant background information, current BSC medical policy, the procedure itself, a review of the scientific literature in reference to the five BCBSA criteria (see Table 2.1), views of pertinent medical societies, and the conclusions and recommendation of the Medical Director. The recommendation for the given technology or procedure is expressed either as "eligible for coverage" or "investigational." Eligibility for coverage may be restricted to particular indications for use or by certain requirements for the qualifications or experience of providers, or a procedure may require preauthorization. The second notebook includes approximately six to 10 of the most important scientific papers on each of the specific medical procedures being considered.

The Medical Policy Committee meets for three half-day meetings each year, once each in San Francisco and Los Angeles, and rotating the third meeting among Sacramento, Orange County, and San Diego. Meetings are open to the public, including representatives of the print and electronic media, and involve open and often-vigorous discussion of the Medical Director's recommendation by the committee members. The committee may also hear oral testimony by experts on a given procedure or technology. Using a majority rule, it then votes, usually to adopt, often to modify, and sometimes to table the recommendation of the Medical Director.

ECRI

ECRI is a nonprofit research organization established in 1955 as the Emergency Care Research Institute. It refocused its attention on medical technology in 1969, and in 1971, it established the Health Devices Program, essentially an equipment and device evaluation service. Hospitals interested in procurement, safety, operation and maintenance, and general technology management were the primary clientele for this effort. In 1981, the organization established the Technology Assessment program and sought to broaden its evaluations and expand its clientele. This effort's foundation, however, remained the evaluation of medical devices and hospital equipment to support hospital procurement. In the late 1980s and early 1990s, ECRI surveyed the medical directors of third-party insurers, concluded that a market existed for technology assessment directed to these individuals, and initiated its current program, the Health Technology Assessment Information Service.

Currently, ECRI provides services in three areas: health care technology, health care risk and quality management, and health care environmental management. In health care technology, the ECRI catalog (ECRI, 1995) lists various online data services (e.g., ECRInet,

Health Devices Sourcebook, Health Devices Alerts), publications (e.g., *Health Devices, Health Devices Alerts, Health Devices Sourcebook, Health Technology Management*), and services to hospitals (e.g., health devices inspection and preventive maintenance system, equipment management software, health product comparison system, capital equipment procurement advisory service). ECRI's main TA effort, the Health Technology Assessment Information Service, describes itself in its catalog as "a comprehensive service that offers in-depth Custom Reports, database searches, regular newsletters, online services, published summaries, educational seminars, and a telephone hotline."

The entire ECRI organization has slightly more than 225 FTE employees, many of whom hold doctorates in science. Of these, 35–40 analysts and information specialists work in TA. The organization has strict conflict-of-interest policies that are consistently enforced: It accepts no advertising or financial support from medical product manufacturers, and no employee may own stock in or consult for a medical equipment or pharmaceutical company. Staff members working in the Health Technology Assessment Information Service are prohibited from holding investments in managed care organizations and health insurers.

In the past five years, ECRI has increased the number and comprehensiveness of its TAs and now produces about 20–25 annually. Recent custom reports on oncology have included assessment of the use of autologous bone marrow transplantation (ABMT) in the treatment of breast cancer, lung cancer, multiple myeloma, and ovarian cancer; and the use of interleukin-2 (IL-2) for the treatment of malignant melanoma and renal cell carcinoma. Reports on cardiovascular treatments have assessed tissue plasminogen activator (tPA) versus streptokinase for treating acute myocardial infarction and have evaluated left ventricular assist devices (LVADs). A large number of assessments of general medical devices, e.g., continuous lumbar passive motion devices for postoperative back surgery, and of imaging devices, e.g., ionic versus nonionic radiographic contrast media, also are performed.

The customers for ECRI's TA service include hospitals; physician organizations; the medical directors of corporate health plans, HMOs, and other managed care organizations; health insurers; and

CHAMPUS, HCFA, and some state governments, e.g., Tennessee. In addition, health care executives are a market for summaries of longer reports. A variety of arrangements is available for purchasing ECRI technology assessment reports and other services. Under one of these arrangements, a subscription to ECRI's technology assessment service costs $15,000 per year, for which a subscriber gets six off-the-shelf reports and may request two new reports specific to its own needs. That subscribers can request customized TAs makes ECRI attractive to some parties.

In its work for public and private payers, ECRI stresses the separation of technology assessment from coverage decisionmaking. It believes that the former process is an objective evaluation of clinical and scientific evidence, whereas the latter is embedded in business, contractual, or regulatory considerations. In this way, ECRI seeks to ensure that its TA services bear scrutiny for technical merit and to avoid financial and intellectual conflicts of interest. The organization's reports and processes are reviewed by an external audit committee of experts, from both public and private sectors, who are committed to independent technology assessment and serve in an unpaid capacity.

NEW (OR NEWLY VISIBLE) TA ORGANIZATIONS

Evidence of increased demand for technology assessment has become apparent with the emergence in the past decade of new organizational performers of TAs. These newer entrants may be established organizations with a new TA effort, or they may be new TA organizations. They constitute a response to the changing health-care marketplace.

In this section, we consider Aetna, Group Health Cooperative of Puget Sound, Harvard Community Health Plan, HAYES, the Institute for Clinical Systems Integration, Kaiser-Permanente Medical Group, Kaiser-Permanente Southern California, Kaiser-Permanente Northern California, Prudential, TEMINEX, United HealthCare, and University HealthSystem Consortium.

Aetna[1]

Aetna has 21,000 employees and about 18 million covered lives, 15 million of whom are in health plans. Its products include traditional indemnity insurance (2–2.5 million policyholders); point-of-service plans, which offer individuals a choice of service at the time the service is sought, rather than at enrollment (3.5 million covered lives and growing rapidly); HMOs (2 million covered lives); and PPOs (4 million covered lives). Aetna's national policy covers 24 HMOs. (See Weiner and deLissovoy, 1993, pp. 94–101, for a glossary of managed care terms.)

Technology assessment is housed organizationally under Clinical and Coverage Policy (CCP), which also includes practice guidelines, clinical decision support, and the Institutes of Excellence network for organ and bone marrow transplantation. In addition, CCP has developed a cardiac care network. The TA unit consists of four physicians, one Ph.D., and three R.N.s. It develops outcomes-based evaluations and precertification protocols for high-volume procedures that have a potential for high cost and controversy. The clinical-decision support group includes two medical librarians, who respond to 6,000 queries each year, and a nurse who responds to field inquiries full-time.

Technology assessment provides direct support for coverage decisions. Assessments include, for example, peripheral endovascular interventions (peripheral laser-assisted angioplasty, peripheral atherectomy, peripheral intraluminal stent placement), ambulatory event (transtelephonic) monitoring, and use of high-dose chemotherapy and bone marrow/peripheral stem cell transplant for Hodgkin's disease. As of April 1996, Aetna had 315 assessments and policies online (through Med Query, its electronic information service) for immediate access by its employees and health plan medical directors. Assessments also provide the precertification criteria for utilization management for HMOs and PPOs, including the patient-selection criteria.

An assessment focuses on the indications for use of a technology and the data in the literature that support those indications. It includes

---

[1]This information was obtained in 1995, before Aetna purchased U.S. HealthCare.

sections on clinical policy, the disease or disorder, and outcome data. Evidence tables containing patient outcome data are included in major assessments, but not in the 2–3-page smaller assessments. A draft TA is reviewed by the Medical Directors' Advisory Committee, and the Policy Review group (for business, legal, and actuarial aspects). The director of TA prepares the final TA. An assessment is then incorporated into a coverage policy document, which also takes federal and state coverage mandates into account, as well as provisions stipulated by the customer.

TA is entirely internal to Aetna, which does not subscribe to BCBSA or ECRI. Turnaround time for an assessment is eight weeks. Volume for 1993 was 45 major TAs and 55 smaller assessments; for 1994, it was 30–35 and 40–50, respectively; and for 1995, 40–45 and 40–50, respectively.

Aetna's TA program is limited to devices and procedures. It emphasizes new technologies; however, policies for existing technologies are reviewed and updated; and some widely accepted procedures for which there are no effectiveness data are occasionally reviewed. Assessments for drugs are handled by Aetna Pharmacy Management, a separate subsidiary. (For coordination between drugs and devices, the head of CCP chairs the Aetna Pharmacy and Therapeutics Committee.) This organization reviews FDA-approved drugs, which usually involves automatic approval for indemnity and PPO plans; reviews off-label uses (i.e., for any, rather than for a specific, indication; see Chapter Three subsection "Off-Label Uses of Approved Drugs"); and manages the drug formulary for the Aetna HMOs. Managing the HMO drug formulary involves analyzing the effectiveness of a new drug and its cost relative to those for drugs already in the formulary, and sometimes cost-effectiveness—the only place in the Aetna system where cost is examined in direct relation to clinical outcomes for purposes of coverage.

Aetna established a terminal-illness procedure five years ago, providing the stimulus for the Medical Care Ombudsman Program (MCOP), in Bethesda, Maryland, which handles mostly cancer patients. MCOP's creation was driven by the controversy over the use of high-dose chemotherapy with autologous bone marrow transplantation. When an Aetna HMO medical director disagrees with a physician or patient about the appropriateness of a treatment that has been designated by the National Institutes of Health or by the National Cancer Institute (NCI) for Phase III clinical trial,[2] such as a bone marrow transplant, Aetna does not deny such a case but sends it to MCOP.   A three-physician team reviews the appropriateness of treatment for the particular patient. A Yes vote for treatment by only one of the three reviewers is enough for Aetna to positively decide to cover the procedure. However, the physicians agree in advance that if they unanimously conclude that treatment is not appropriate, they are prepared to go to court to defend their review.   One hundred corporate firms now use MCOP, which is described in Chapter Four.

Group Health Cooperative of Puget Sound

Group Health Cooperative (GHC) of Puget Sound is one of the country's oldest staff-model health maintenance organizations; physicians are salaried employees of the organization. GHC provides services to approximately 480,000 members in three geographic regions of western Washington. Under the aegis of GHC Clinical Planning and Improvement, three long-standing committees—the Committee on Medically Emerging Technologies (COMET), the Pharmacy and Therapeutics Committee (P&T), and the Committee on Prevention (COP)—manage GHC's technology assessment and practice guidelines efforts.

COMET, established in 1981, evaluates new medical procedures, devices, and practices. The committee conducts secondary TAs based on available data and on the credibility of the data source. The evaluation criteria are reliability and safety, health outcomes, satisfaction and desirability, and cost. Health outcomes are either primary end points or secondary end points that have a defined relationship to primary end points. Costs are assessed in relation to existing options, if any; but, reportedly, other criteria besides cost dominate decisions. The results of an assessment, then, are that a technology is "clearly effective," "clearly ineffective," or "of indeterminate effectiveness."

------

[2]In Phase I trials, safety and pharmacological profiling in humans is tested; Phase II trials involve initial testing of effectiveness in humans; and Phase III trials involve extensive clinical trials of effectiveness in humans.

When existing data are unclear or inadequate, resulting in an "indeterminate effectiveness" judgment, GHC often institutes an internal clinical trial, in which data are collected by its physicians in accordance with a protocol and results are reported back to the committee periodically. For example, visually assisted laser prostatectomy, an outpatient procedure, was considered by COMET. GHC urologists, strongly supported by device manufacturers, were promoting the procedure's use. Because the data about outcomes were poor or nonexistent, a trial was designed, with assistance from the Center for Health Studies (GHC's health services research unit), and data were collected at 3, 6, 9, and 12 months. At 12 months, 100 patients had received the treatment: When these patients were matched against the controls, who had received transurethral prostatectomy, the outcomes were the same for both groups. The costs of the new procedure were substantially less than surgical prostatectomy; however, in the period after the procedure, treated patients reported more burning, bleeding, and pain. GHC decided that these data should be shared with patients, even though it was not in its immediate financial interest to do so.

The P&T Committee is more than 20 years old and has primary responsibility for managing the GHC formulary. In recent years, it has shifted from consensus-based to evidence-based assessments of new drugs for supporting formulary decisions. One procedural change is that the P&T Committee no longer allows requests for adding a new drug to come from an individual physician; instead, it requires that requests come from GHC divisions and that they be supported by data from the pertinent scientific literature. If an assessment of a new drug is favorable on effectiveness grounds, and the drug's cost to GHC is estimated at less than $50,000 a year, the committee has authority to decide for the organization; if GHC's estimated outlay is greater than $50,000, the committee forwards its recommendation to the GHC Executive Council for decision. A rough form of cost-effectiveness analysis—cost-minimization—is done, whereby the costs of comparable therapeutic agents are compared. Increasingly, the P&T Committee compares the costs of the drug to the costs of no drug and the associated sequelae, such as hospitalization.

The P&T Committee confronts several challenges. It follows the FDA docket closely for drug approvals, especially for those with a big political or financial effect, such as RU 486, an abortion-inducing medication for which there is strong demand and to which there is great opposition. But there is substantial pressure on the FDA to review more drugs, such as those for treating cancer or AIDS, on a fast-track, or accelerated-approval, basis, basing approvals on surrogate end points (or nonclinical proxies for the usual required data about clinical outcomes). This, in turn, makes evidence-based assessment of patient benefit by GHC, and other health plans, more difficult. Another challenge to the committee is to shift the balance of its energies from formulary management, a continuing responsibility, to influencing physicians' prescribing behavior. This objective is being helped by the installation of a computerized prescription-order-entry system, which will allow prescription data to be integrated with the diagnosis of a patient's disease or condition and, eventually, with a protocol for disease management.

The Committee on Prevention is oriented to primary and secondary prevention. Priorities for COP topic selection are based on the criteria that (1) a clinical condition has a significant mortality, morbidity, or cost; (2) the condition is pre-symptomatic; (3) the condition is detectable; (4) an effective intervention exists; (5) GHC has the capacity to address the problem; and (6) resource use is justified on cost-effectiveness grounds. The eleven key GHC prevention areas include tobacco use, cervical cancer, breast cancer, and HIV.

Until this past year, a fourth committee was involved, the Committee on Practice Efficacy (COPE), which was the clinical practice guidelines committee. COPE addressed the management of a disease entity or clinical condition, often with respect to a defined patient population, in contrast to the COMET and P&T focus on specific technologies. It based its priorities on the identification of a gap between high-quality literature and internal GHC data—i.e., if the data in the literature or within GHC were good, no guideline was developed; if the data were inadequate and the problem was important, a guideline would be developed. COPE has now been absorbed into a corporate oversight committee that helps divisions within GHC by providing them with a model of the criteria and processes for guidelines development.

Two characteristics of GHC guidelines are worth noting. First, a guideline is based on a careful assessment of the data in the scientific literature. Second, a good deal of attention is given to implementation of the guideline (Handley et al., 1994). For example, in April 1991, a paper appearing in the *New England Journal of Medicine* (Catalona et al., 1991) stated that prostate-specific antigen (PSA) testing "identifies patients at high risk for prostate cancer." The result at GHC was that PSA test ordering jumped from 250 tests per month to 700. This result prompted financial concern, as well as physician unease about using the test for screening purposes. A quick literature review led to the conclusion that PSA testing did not meet standard criteria for an acceptable screening test and that the clinical decisions made in response to test results might increase mortality and morbidity (Stuart et al., 1992).

Consequently, in early 1995, GHC published a guideline, *Prostate Specific Antigen (PSA) As a Screening Test for Prostate Cancer,* for its physicians and patients (GHCPS, 1995), using internal GHC data developed in the interim. (The guideline had been preceded by two papers, one in *HMO Practice* [Stuart et al., 1992] and another in the *Journal of Urology* [Handley and Stuart, 1994]; the latter reported a marked reduction in PSA tests in the feedback period following the assessment.) The guideline "Evidence Summary" for physicians included background information about prostate cancer and data on PSA test characteristics (low sensitivity, ~70–80 percent; low specificity, ~38–59 percent; and low positive predictive value, ~10–50 percent).

A discussion of benefits noted the absence of randomized-clinical-trial data showing that early detection of prostate cancer results in a decrease in cancer-specific mortality. The summary also discussed the risks of the "cascade of interventions" that often were triggered by a positive PSA test result, including those associated with radical prostatectomy and radiation therapy. It concluded that "insufficient evidence" existed to support the use of PSA as a beneficial screening test for prostate cancer but that the test was of "known usefulness in monitoring the response to treatment of patients with known prostate cancer."

The two-sided single sheet of patient information reviews the facts about prostate cancer, the two detection methods (digital rectal examination, PSA test), some facts about the PSA test, and the implications of a positive PSA test result for treatment options (i.e., watchful waiting, radiation treatment, surgery, male hormone therapy), including the risks of each treatment (e.g., impotence, incontinence, death).

Four factors highlight the commitment of GHC to using TA as an integral element in its management of the health care it delivers. First, the commitment to evidence-based TAs, P&T decisions, guidelines (including prevention guidelines), and to clinical care in general, appears to be genuine and deep. Dr. Michael Stuart, who had been the COPE chairman, and Dr. Matthew Handley have developed an instructional manual, *An Evidence-Based Approach to Changing Clinical Practice* (Stuart and Handley, n.d.), that has been widely used in GHC's own continuing-education program. Second, the Division of Clinical Planning and Improvement is now seeking to integrate its historically independent TA and guidelines committees at points of commonality; e.g., all groups now use the same format for evidence tables. Third, the Center for Health Studies, the GHC health services research arm, supports clinical planning and improvement efforts in a number of ways, for example, by participating in the design of studies undertaken by the several committees. Fourth, substantial investments in data systems augur an even stronger capability than currently exists to generate internal data on clinical effectiveness, patient outcomes, patient satisfaction, and cost.

Harvard Community Health Plan[3]

The Harvard Community Health Plan (HCHP) is an HMO with 570,000 enrolled members. Its Clinical Quality Management Department, which is oriented to health outcomes and clinical planning and improvement, oversees technology assessments *and* clinical practice guidelines. Both TAs and guidelines use many of the same evidence-based processes, but guidelines are concerned with processes of care and with managing clinical conditions. (TA is sometimes referred to as a *single-mode guideline*.)

TAs are the province of the Committee for Appropriate Technology (CAT), which was organized in June 1992. The CAT, which meets

---

[3]This discussion is based on information that was obtained before the merger of HCHP and Pilgrim Health System, now Harvard-Pilgrim HealthCare.

every other month, is made up of senior clinical leaders of HCHP (the Associate Medical Director for Clinical Quality, the medical directors of HCHP's three divisions, the Chief of Surgical Specialties, the Associate Medical Director for Practice Systems), the director of benefits and contracts for the Health Centers Division, the TA program manager, and a representative of the Fertility Review Board.

The CAT is a policymaking board for HCHP. It generally does not deal with specific cases; for external expert review on specific cases, it often contracts with the Medical Care Ombudsman Program (see Chapter Four for a discussion of MCOP). Rather, it considers safety and efficacy, legal issues, marketing, adverse-selection effects,[4] and ethical aspects of the primarily new technologies it reviews. It also reviews new indications and appropriate uses for existing technologies. An example of one of the technologies assessed is pallidotomy for the treatment of Parkinson's disease.

The TA process is as follows: For a given topic, an expert panel of physicians, mainly from HCHP but including outside experts if necessary, is established to conduct the assessment. Members of the panel conduct an evidence-based literature review and prepare evidence tables. The entire panel reviews the evidence and makes recommendations to the CAT about the safety, efficacy, clinical effectiveness, and cost-effectiveness of the technology. Those recommendations are presented to the CAT by a clinician from the expert panel, whenever possible, and the TA manager. The CAT then writes draft policies based on the evidence and rationale derived from the assessments. Draft policies are sent to approximately 120 HCHP clinical managers for review and may go through several revisions, depending on the comments received. The TA manager synthesizes the comments; if major clinical issues are raised, however, the literature is reexamined and the matter may be referred again to the expert panel. On completion of this process, the CAT issues policies.

---

[4]In this context, adverse-selection effects occur when the decision of one health plan to cover a new technology or procedure is not followed by other plans, and the plan attracts to its membership a disproportionate number of individuals who expect to benefit from that decision, thus adversely affecting the health plan and its financial situation.

The HCHP TA level of effort is modest: 1.0 –1.5 FTE staff support. It relies mainly on its own physicians for conducting TAs, but often brings in specialists affiliated with contract or partner hospitals, such as Brigham and Women's Hospital and Massachusetts General Hospital. In addition, as a member of The HMO Group, HCHP uses its TEMINEX service,[5] often for short-turnaround assessments, and has informal access to the medical directors of other HMO Group member plans. HCHP also subscribes to ECRI's service, partly for customized reports.

HAYES, Inc.

In 1989, Dr. Winifred Hayes, a consultant to health insurers, concluded that a market existed in the payer community for TA support of health coverage decisions, and incorporated HAYES, Inc., a consulting services organization, with both a managed care and workers' compensation focus. ECRI had not yet entered the payer market, BCBSA's assessments were still limited to member plans, and significant TA capability within the insurance industry was limited mainly to large insurers, such as Aetna and Prudential. Likewise, the number and timeliness of assessments produced by the federal government through OHTA and OTA did not meet private-sector needs. HAYES expected its initial market to be senior claims analysts in small to mid-sized insurance companies and HMOs. As it has turned out, however, most users are physicians, nurses, attorneys, and senior managers dealing with claims and contract issues. Customers include a number of large HMOs, insurance carriers, PPOs, and the states of Minnesota and Tennessee.

HAYES published its first TA report in March 1991 and now markets two TA-related services: *The HAYES Directory of New Medical Technologies' Status* and *The HAYES Directory of Legal Precedent Reports.*

The Hayes Directory of New Medical Technologies' Status is a series of assessment reports on drugs, biologicals, devices, diagnostic tests, and medical and surgical procedures. As of December 1995, this di-

---

[5]TEMINEX (Technology Management Information Exchange) is a service to the medical directors of The HMO Group member plans. It is described below.

rectory comprised eight volumes and about 450 reports. Existing reports are updated periodically; new reports are added quarterly. At present, two-thirds or more of the 20–30 reports issued each quarter are updates of existing reports. HAYES' reports are based on information available in the published scientific literature, along with data from federal agencies and professional societies, including NIH consensus conference statements, HCFA coverage decisions, FDA decisions, and position statements and guidelines developed by medical-specialty societies and associations such as the American College of Physicians, the American College of Obstetrics and Gynecology, and the American Medical Association. Reports deal with safety, efficacy, patient-selection criteria, effect of technologies on health outcomes, comparisons with alternative technologies, and cost.

The second product line is the recently introduced *HAYES Directory of Legal Precedent Reports.* These reports deal with medical technologies that involve controversial legal issues pertaining to both medical malpractice and claims coverage litigation. The approximately 10 reports produced quarterly review and discuss the emergence of case precedents, regulations, and statutes that apply to technologies and issues.

The organization has also begun to enter the hospital market. Its hospital-related reports focus on the acquisition of new technology; however, rather than medical device performance, the focus of these reports is on risk management, quality assurance, utilization review, and the effect of technology on health outcomes. HAYES' reports are available online through West Publishing (Westlaw) and, in early 1996, through Reed Elsevier (Lexis-Nexis).

In its medical technology assessments, HAYES does not use unpublished research data (sometimes called the "gray literature"), except on a customized basis for a specific client, but generally relies instead on the peer-reviewed journal literature. Also, as a precaution against expert bias, HAYES avoids using specialty panels of experts to routinely review its products. Instead, HAYES uses a panel of physician-generalists with specialist training for advice on coverage decisions and practice guidelines, incorporating both evidence-based TAs and expert opinion in its review and recommendations regarding the care of specific patients, policy development, and practice guidelines development.

The HAYES staff consists of 7 full-time and 7 part-time employees, and 20 individual contractors (who may work as much as 20–30 hours per week for HAYES), most of whom are medical writers and editors, with varied medical backgrounds. The Philadelphia area, with its many pharmaceutical firms, is rich in freelance medical writers. No M.D.s are currently used as primary writers; however, physicians with research training are used as medical editors, evaluating the evidence by reading for content accuracy, completeness, and relevancy.

Detailed information about pricing of the HAYES service—the *Directory* and the quarterly updates—is proprietary. In general, the organization wishes customers to use its entire service, not just single reports. Pricing for a health plan, for example, is a function of the number of employees covered under the plan, the number of locations at which the service will be used, and the form in which the information is provided: For a small Taft-Hartley plan with 5,000 members, the initial cost may be $2,000 and the annual fee, an additional $1,000. For a large, multi-plan managed care organization, the cost may exceed $100,000 per year.

Institute for Clinical Systems Integration

The Institute for Clinical Systems Integration (ICSI) originated in response to a Request for Proposals (RFP) issued in February 1992 by the Business Health Care Action Group, a coalition of major Minneapolis–St. Paul employers, to health care providers (see Chapter One). Among other things, the RFP called for a capability to measure quality and outcomes and to conduct technology assessments. The award-winning response came from GroupCare Consortium, which comprised Group Health, Inc., and its affiliated clinics, MedCenters Health Plan, the Mayo Clinic, and Park Nicollet Medical Center. (Group Health and MedCenters merged in 1992 to form HealthPartners, which absorbed Ramsey Hospital and Clinic in 1993.) The winning proposal led to the creation of ICSI as an entity for developing clinical practice guidelines and technology assessments.

ICSI, established in 1993, is a 501(c)(3) nonprofit organization whose founding members are HealthPartners, Mayo, and Park Nicollet. Other participating organizations include 17 smaller Minnesota medical groups. The ICSI board includes three representatives from HealthPartners, two from Mayo, three from Park Nicollet, two physicians from other medical groups, and three purchasers, including one from the BHCAG. Each year, HealthPartners pays $1.8 million to ICSI, which has a staff of 12, of whom 8 are professionals. The participating medical groups contribute in-kind services (basically, physician time) to guidelines development and TA efforts; the total annual contribution is estimated at $3–$4 million from all groups, with Mayo and Park Nicollet each providing approximately $800,000 of this amount per year.

The above arrangement means that ICSI is controlled by physicians from the medical groups but is funded by HealthPartners, the HMO, a design intended to separate the preparation of guidelines and the conduct of TAs from decisions that the health plan must make on benefits and benefit design issues. ICSI reports go to the HMO as inputs to plan decisionmaking.

ICSI identifies six areas of long-term effort: *population health*—the general health status and health risk behaviors of specific populations; guidelines development (see below); measurement—of the effectiveness and appropriateness of practices in relation to guidelines and outcomes; technology assessment (see below); automation of clinical information; and continuous quality improvement. The guidelines-development process is described as follows (ICSI, 1995):

> the process of analyzing all possible ways of treating a particular
> health condition to discover the current best practice. A guideline
> for care is then established in the participating medical groups so
> that all patients will receive the same high quality of care with little
> variation regardless of the individual physician's practice style or
> geographic location.

The process of guidelines development involves, first, that a topic be selected on the bases of health conditions common to a population, the potential effect of guidelines on that condition, the feasibility of developing and implementing guidelines, and the cost and frequency of treatment for that condition. Next, a guideline work group of cross-disciplinary experts is established to examine various treatment approaches and the associated outcomes data; identify the treatment that "yields the best, most consistent outcomes"; and draft a guideline, with rationale and references, and measurement specifications for implementation. The draft guideline is then distributed for systemwide review, re-drafted in response to comments, pilot-tested, and then implemented on a systemwide basis. Once implemented, a guideline is periodically reviewed and monitored. Guidelines development is the primary ICSI activity.

TA is important but has a slightly different focus from guidelines and occurs at a somewhat earlier stage of development. ICSI (1995) describes technology assessment as

> the evaluation of new medical technology for its effectiveness. The results of technology assessment are incorporated into health care guidelines so that purchasers and patients will have the prompt benefit of new and effective technology and will not be subject to unnecessary costs due to the use of ineffective technology.

TAs are supported by one full-time ICSI staff member and are organized under a Technology Assessment Committee (Stecher et al., 1995). Committee members are appointed by ICSI and represent the various research and primary- and specialty-care medical departments from the participating medical groups; the chair of the HealthPartners Benefits committee and a representative of BHCAG are also members.

When a specific TA is undertaken, a work group is formed of experts in clinical medicine, epidemiology, and study-design competence. A given assessment focuses narrowly on a specific new technology or procedure and is intended to aid clinicians in participating medical groups and to support coverage decisions of HealthPartners. The same evidence-based criteria that are used for guidelines are used for TAs. However, adequate data are seldom available for review; therefore, the process depends more on the expert knowledge of work-group members. The evaluation criteria are essentially borrowed from BCBSA. Reports from groups such as TEMINEX, AHCPR, ECRI, and the AMA's DATTA may be used in the TA process.

The TA process does not yet have the same structure as the guidelines-development process. A formal process designed in ICSI's early days was judged too complicated; the organization is currently designing a simpler process.

Kaiser-Permanente Medical Care Program

With 6.5 million members, Kaiser-Permanente is the country's largest and oldest health maintenance organization. It is organized into 12 regions, which by design have a relatively high degree of autonomy from the corporate center, which is located in Oakland, California. Two regions—Northern California and Southern California—account for 2.5 million and 2.2 million members, respectively, or 38 and 34 percent of total members.

At the corporate level, an Inter-Regional New Technologies Committee has been functioning since the mid-1980s. This committee, whose members are drawn from all 12 regions, meets four times a year. At each meeting, it reviews 3–6 technologies or procedures. However, it has conducted over 450 reviews during its decade-long existence. Following a review, the committee *advises* the regions of the views of clinical-expert groups concerning experimental technologies, so that information can be coordinated among the Kaiser regions. Coverage-policy decisionmaking authority and responsibility remain at the regional level.

The New Technologies Committee is supported by one FTE professional and relies heavily on contributed time from regional medical directors and expert physicians on an ad hoc basis for a given assessment. Kaiser-Permanente subscribes to ECRI, receives BCBSA assessments as a result of its relationship with that organization (discussed earlier in this chapter), and also obtains TEMINEX reports. It is prepared to use assessments from any legitimate source.

The New Technologies Committee's work began with the review of medical devices but, when AIDS emerged, its scope was expanded to include drugs. Although the primary review of drugs occurs at the level of the regional P&T committees, drug reviews are coordinated for the New Technologies Committee by one of its members. Although the emphasis of the committee's work is on new technologies, it also re-reviews prior assessments as new information becomes available. Over 100 technologies that were previously judged "experimental" have been reevaluated.

Designating procedures as "experimental" as a basis for coverage decisionmaking, which has been traditional in health insurance, is losing its usefulness within health care generally and within Kaiser specifically. As Dr. Ian Leverton, Director of Permanente Inter-Regional Services, said, "'Experimental' doesn't help in court. Any definition is problematic. A roomful of lawyers working for a week cannot write a definition" (telephone interview, October 4, 1995). Among the Kaiser regions, especially Kaiser-Permanente of Northern California, the emerging alternative is to push the coverage decision down to the individual physician and individual patient, where the focus becomes the medical appropriateness of care.

At the level of the Inter-Regional Committee, deliberations and judgments about technologies and procedures rely heavily on the scientific literature for data about clinical efficacy. Consequently, the fact that randomized clinical trials are becoming more difficult to conduct has become cause for concern. In particular, the ethical constraints to double-blind clinical trials, the soundest methodological approach for determining medical efficacy, have become more severe. In addition, patient preferences for new procedures, physician advocacy, and manufacturers' interests in shorter trials are all factors limiting the ability to perform good trials. Given the dependence of TA on the published literature, this issue is seen within Kaiser as troublesome and is becoming more so.

Cost-effectiveness is not a major part of Kaiser-Permanente assessments. A spokesman indicated that the New Technologies Committee had not conducted cost-effectiveness analyses of procedures, but was "pure and virginal" in that regard (telephone interview with Ian Leverton, M.D., October 4, 1995). Although expressing the view that cost-effectiveness assessment (CEA) was an appropriate direction in which to move, he noted that then-existing Kaiser data systems at the corporate level did not permit such analyses to be done.

In general, the significant technology assessments within the Kaiser system are done by the regions, which strongly influence the work of the Inter-Regional Committee. We focus, then, on the two largest regions, Kaiser-Permanente of Southern California and Kaiser-Permanente of Northern California.

Kaiser-Permanente of Southern California

Kaiser-Permanente of Southern California (KPSC) is organized into 11 subregional areas, has 3,000 physicians, owns 10 hospitals, and has 2.2 million members. In mid-1995, it merged its existing technology assessment and clinical practice guidelines efforts into a new Department of Clinical Analysis, marking the end of an internal evolutionary stage of technology management and assessment.

A long-standing KPSC Medical Technology Committee has been concerned with the acquisition of capital equipment and its associated logistics. That function is now supported by the Department of Clinical Analysis, whose assessments address appropriate utilization, clinical needs of provider and patient, equitable distribution of technologies within the region, and the economics of procurement. Similarly, a long-standing P&T Committee has maintained the formulary at KPSC hospitals, examining the merit of a drug for a selected group of patients—e.g., the use of Tacrine for the amelioration of Alzheimer's disease. This committee is also now supported by the new department.

Given both the dramatic health benefits claimed for biotechnology products before their release and the high cost of such products, a separate Biologicals Committee was established in 1992 to track and evaluate biotechnology products before their approval by FDA. (For example, when beta-interferon was released, no cure existed for multiple sclerosis. Yet the press reported the biologic as a potential cure, generating intense interest among patients and demand for its use by KPSC patients and physicians.) The Biologicals Committee appoints a working group of physicians, pharmacists, and analysts for each biotechnology product as FDA approval approaches and as clinical data become available. After consensus-building within relevant specialty groups, the evidence-based assessments of the Biologicals Committee go as recommendations to the P&T Committee for a formulary decision.

Currently, attention is being given to the implications of genetic technology research for KPSC. Genetics poses a challenge for evaluation: A number of genetic tests are on the market for conditions for which no treatment exists; consequently, many ethical issues surround the use of such tests. Some of the KPSC effort in this area is directed to the education of the primary-care physician. Interest in genetics was initiated by the KPSC Biologicals Committee, but has now migrated to an independent interregional project team examining BRCA-1 (a genetic marker predictive of breast cancer in some women) in an effort to develop a clinical practice guideline.

Clinical practice guidelines are at the heart of the KPSC technology assessment of procedures. Efforts focus on those key areas of medical practice identified by KP physicians in which *best practice* can be defined and implemented. Assessments are conducted by physicians and TA analysts through existing groups of medical-specialty chiefs, regional committees, transplant committees, and ad hoc task forces. Evidence-based assessments involve extensive review of the efficacy of clinical interventions. Health policies result from those assessments, and their implementation is monitored for health outcomes and utilization on an ongoing basis. Policies are reviewed periodically as new scientific evidence and monitoring data become available.

Kaiser-Permanente of Northern California

Kaiser-Permanente of Northern California (KPNC), the largest of the 12 Kaiser regions, has 3,500 physicians, owns 15 hospitals, and has 2.5 million enrollees. For its TA activity, KPNC relies heavily on BCBSA determinations about when, on the basis of the published scientific literature, a technology is no longer "investigational." It also subscribes to ECRI. Infrequently, it will conduct an assessment itself, typically when none has been done by another organization. For example, it reviewed 4–5 procedures in 1994 that no one else, to its knowledge, had assessed, including 3-marker screening for genetic defects, small-bowel nutrition (for taking small-bowel patients off total parenteral nutrition), and cryoprostatectomy (for which a specific case required an evaluation).

KPNC's evaluation of medical technology, however, emphasizes the provision of medically appropriate treatment to its enrollees. Consequently, most of its activity focuses on the review of cases of individual patients who, with their physician, are considering a treatment for which inadequate evidence of safety and efficacy exists. Such situations occur when a disease is very rare or when the difference in benefit between two treatments is so small that a definitive clinical trial would require large numbers of patients and many years of data collection. In contrast to the few formal assessments it conducts, KPNC reviews many individual-patient cases. For example, in 1994, single-case reviews of transplantation were estimated at 80 bone marrow transplants, 50 liver transplants, and about 40 heart transplants.

Case reviews are conducted by Permanente Medical Group physicians who are expert in a particular clinical area. KPNC has about 15 standing clinical groups, or councils, which are built around a medical specialty or several related specialties. These councils meet regularly and may have a technology subgroup. For example, the bone-marrow-transplant council is made up of adult and pediatric oncologists and hematologists, and has a subgroup for technologies. These councils have the primary responsibility for reviewing whether a particular treatment should be offered to a given patient. The process is based on the consensus of experts about cases involving treatments for which no evidence of efficacy or effectiveness yet exists.

If a KPNC clinical group decides that treatment for a given patient is medically appropriate even though experimental, referral of the patient for enrollment in a clinical trial is provided. These referrals are based on standing agreements with major medical centers, such as Stanford. If the decision is to deny treatment, however, a three-level appeals process is available for the patient who disagrees with the judgment: The first-level appeal goes to the advisory council; the second appeal goes to two Kaiser physicians not involved with the case; and the third goes to the Medical Care Ombudsman Program of Bethesda, Maryland, which maintains a national roster of physicians for responding to such appeals (see Chapter Four for more detail).

KPNC has moved away from denial of coverage for experimental treatments, currently allowing patients to receive experimental treatments if they enroll in a clinical trial. In 1996, it planned to remove the exclusionary language on experimental treatments from its contracts. The critical issue for KPNC is no longer exclusionary contract language but medical appropriateness as determined by expert physician review.

Other evaluative tasks are performed by different groups. P&T committees at each medical center are overseen by a regional group; their job is to maintain the formulary. Medical device acquisition is handled by some 25 groups—e.g., for patient monitoring, imaging, nuclear medicine, intensive-care nursery—made up of clinicians, biomedical engineers, and others. These groups review devices, visit manufacturers, and review internal data, then enter into an exclusive contract with a single manufacturer for all Northern California medical groups. On the basis of this work, interregional contracts are now being developed for many products within the overall Kaiser system.

KPNC does not conduct cost-effectiveness analyses of new technologies; rather, its cost analyses are oriented toward management decisions: whether a given capability should be provided directly by Kaiser-Permanente or should be obtained on a contract basis (the "make-or-buy" decision). A spokesman noted that a widespread public impression and frequent criticism of HMOs is that they have financial incentives to undertreat patients. This criticism, he continued, constitutes a disincentive to do formal cost-effectiveness analysis, which spokesmen suggest would only reinforce a negative public image. This is a decidedly different limitation on cost-effectiveness analysis from the data limitation identified by the Kaiser corporate spokesman in the preceding subsection.

KPNC differs substantially at present from KPSC. The contrast between these two regions, which together include more than 80 percent of all Kaiser members, suggests some of the limits of TA as well as different strategies for dealing with new technology.

Prudential

Prudential is a national insurance company. Its 50–55 local health plans are defined geographically by cities and are grouped in five regions. Local plans have a relatively high degree of autonomy. The company business includes both traditional indemnity health insurance and managed care products.

To ensure uniformity and efficiency among its member plans, the Prudential home office has operated a formal TA program since 1985. The TA program supports two types of organizational decisions: corporate policies on coverage to guide local plans, and case-by-case decisions by local-plan medical directors on preauthorization, and sometimes after-the-fact authorization, of treatments.

The Prudential TA effort is staffed by approximately 10 professionals, primarily nurses and individuals with insurance experience, who conduct about 40–45 TAs each year. The criteria for assessing a technology include the following:

- The technology involves a new method of preventing, diagnosing, or treating a health problem.

- It involves a service that is frequently utilized, or costly, or controversial, or subject to rapid change, or subject to fraud and abuse practices.

- New data have become available.

- A given Medical Technical Evaluation and Coverage Statement (M-TECS; see description below) has not been reviewed in the past three years.

Assessments involve review of the peer-reviewed literature, official statements of professional medical-specialty societies, consensus statements from government agencies, TAs performed by public and private agencies, and policies of federal agencies (e.g., FDA, NIH, AHCPR, HCFA). Staff select the pertinent studies, summarize the results of those studies, and formulate conclusions in a draft assessment. Draft assessments are then reviewed by the medical leadership of Prudential, are sent to 70–80 physician consultants for review and comment, and are then distributed to the five regions.

The final review of a draft TA is done by the Technology Assessment Advisory Committee (TAAC), which meets quarterly and includes corporate representatives from Underwriting, Claims Management, Executive Management, Pharmacy, Marketing, Contracts, Medical, and Legal. The TAAC has final authority to approve an assessment, which is issued as a Medical Technology Evaluation and Coverage Statement, a three-part document consisting of a claim-administration summary, a clinical summary, and the longer assessment. The claim summary and full assessment are proprietary and are distributed only within Prudential; the clinical summary is sometimes distributed to, among others, medical personnel of affiliated medical groups. An approved M-TECS is published and distributed to the five Prudential regions, which are responsible for implementing these policies uniformly.

An estimated one-third of the TAs are new; two-thirds are updates of existing policies. Prescription drugs are reviewed by a separate pharmacy benefits unit. An estimated one-third of the drugs reviewed are newly approved agents, and about two-thirds involve off-label use of FDA-approved drugs.

Prudential subscribes to the BCBSA TA service and attends its Medical Advisory Panel meetings, and also subscribes to ECRI's service, to the AMA's DATTA, and, according to one officer, to "whatever is out there."

Prudential's evaluative activities go beyond technology assessment and include related health-services research and practice-guidelines development. In 1993, when Dr. William L. Roper, former Administrator of the Health Care Financing Administration and former Director of the Centers for Disease Control, joined the company as Vice President, he established what is now known as the Prudential Center for Health Services Research. Staffed by over 20 individuals, the Center has 25 health-outcomes studies under way that are intended to support the 5 million Prudential enrollees. Prudential staff conduct studies that deal with, for example, the improvement of immunization rates, the improvement of mammography rates, and guidelines for treating low-back pain and for managing diabetes. The first studies are now being completed; the results are being submitted to peer-reviewed journals so that they may be widely available to the public. Clinical practice guidelines are also being developed at the local health-plan level, with guidance from the Prudential corporate offices. Some studies are also done, on a contract basis, by the Department of Health Care Policy of Harvard Medical School.

TEMINEX (of The HMO Group)

The HMO Group was established in 1984. As of January 1, 1995, the 30 member and associate member plans constituting the Group were serving more than 7 million members. The major plans include Kaiser-Permanente, nine of whose regions joined in 1994; Group Health Cooperative of Puget Sound; HealthPartners of Minnesota;

Harvard Pilgrim HealthPlan; and Health Insurance Plan of Greater New York. The mission of the organization is to strengthen group-practice HMOs through collaborative activities in affordability, member satisfaction, and improved health status, and to promote group-practice HMOs to purchasers, consumers, regulators, and the public. Its programs include the exchange of data to measure, report, and improve performance of its member plans; the promotion of total quality management systems; the formation of management councils for meetings of senior HMO managers (directors, medical directors, finance directors, marketing directors) to share information; and clinical symposia and technical seminars on issues pertinent to prepaid group practice.

The Technology Management Information Exchange (TEMINEX) is a service to the medical directors of The HMO Group member plans. Located in Buffalo, New York, it employs approximately 2.5 full-time professionals (an M.D. who provides oversight, an M.D.–Ph.D. project manager, and an epidemiologist). On request, TEMINEX staff provide plans with evidence-based secondary assessments of health care technologies. These assessments are advisory to plans, but the plans make decisions. TEMINEX publicly disclaims liability for member-coverage decisions. Plans seek TEMINEX advice on the following: the appropriate use of a health care technology for a specific patient; prospective assessment of a technology's potential effect on a plan[6] and advice on managing that effect; support for a plan's own technology assessment activities; and assistance in clinical guidelines development.

TEMINEX assessments involve a literature review, a rating of the evidence, and compilation of the opinions of key consultants regarding probabilities of success of a procedure, the best treatment centers for performing that procedure, and the best outcomes for a patient. The evidence rating is illustrated by a September 1994 TEMINEX report on intravenous immunoglobulin for the prevention of recurrent infections in pediatric patients. In response to the question, "Does the peer-reviewed medical literature support the use of IVIG in pediatric patients with recurrent infections, particularly *otitis media*

---

[6]*Prospective assessment* is systematic acquisition of data, using a predefined protocol, on use of a technology and the outcomes of that technology as its use occurs.

and sinusitis, who also have evidence of IgG subclass deficiency and/or lack of response to common angina?" the report noted that

> two small randomized clinical trials which used IVIG to treat patients with multiple episodes of *otitis media* or chronic chest symptoms are available. These trials did not report the IgG subclass status of enrolled patients, were not blinded, included very small numbers of patients, and did not report confidence intervals for the treatment effects attributed to IVIG. Therefore, the randomized clinical trial evidence supporting the use of IVIG in this clinical situation cannot be adequately ranked without the help of a formal meta-analysis.
>
> For the specific clinical situation presented by patients with defined IgG subclass deficiencies and/or inability to respond to common antigen, no evidence supporting the administration of IVIG is available from randomized clinical trials. Reports in the literature are confined to nonrandomized historical cohort studies (Level IV evidence) and case series (Level V evidence).

In addition to preparing reports, TEMINEX serves as a clearinghouse for its member plans. TEMINEX staff survey the technology assessment staff at The HMO Group member plans three times a year for work in progress. They are able to use this information to apprise member plans of others who may be researching the same topic, as well as to identify topics of interest to all or most plans. The members also share assessments among themselves.

United HealthCare

United HealthCare was primarily a national managed care organization of about 20 health plans and some small amount of indemnity insurance until July 1995, when it announced its intention to purchase MetraHealth, a joint venture of Metropolitan Life Insurance Co. and Travellers Group.[7] United has a formal TA program, staffed by one FTE professional, as a central-office support function for its local plans. It also obtains four or five TAs annually from its ECRI subscription that meet a standard of impartiality and provide an in-

---

[7]The information in this section was obtained before United HealthCare acquired MetraHealth.

depth treatment of a technology; subscribes to the HAYES service (described above) as a reference tool; subscribes to the DATTA service; receives the assessments of the Clinical Efficacy Assessment Program of the ACP; obtains AHCPR technology assessments and practice guidelines; and monitors the outputs of professional societies.

Over the past three years, the United TA effort has shifted from focusing exclusively on case reviews of single patients to more-comprehensive analyses of technologies, their indications, data about patient benefit, and comparison with alternative technologies. The following are the criteria for determining TA priorities: A high level of controversy prevails within the medical and scientific community about the efficacy of a technology; the cost implications of a technology are significant; a technology has the potential for rapid diffusion; alternative technologies are available; patient safety and health outcomes may be affected; a substantial patient population may be affected; and public and professional demand for a technology may be at a high level.

TAs involve an evidence-based staff review of the literature, with attention to safety, effectiveness, and outcomes. Staff may also query other national organizations for regulatory information, available clinical guidelines, published assessments on the topic in question, and any referrals that may be appropriate. The literature review is then circulated, for discussion, to physicians throughout the country. Their comments are incorporated into a document that is sent to the corporate medical-management team.

The TA review indicates whether a procedure is safe and effective, and is, or is still considered, "experimental" or "unproven." Coverage recommendations are made for each indication of a safe and effective technology. In addition, an accompanying analysis explains why the technology does or does not surpass conventional technology. A statement about competitor policies on a technology may also be included as part of the assessment. Federal and state government mandates for health care, as well as specific health-plan contract language, are reviewed during the process, because they take precedence over the recommendations of the Medical Services Management Team.

The review is sent next to a United HealthCare TA Review Committee, which includes health-plan medical directors and health-service directors, and corporate representatives from Claims, Legal/Contracts, and Indemnity Products departments. The committee reviews the draft TA and its conclusions. Their comments and the draft then go to the Medical Services Management Team for a final conclusion and preparation of the assessment for distribution to member plans with the next *Medical Management Manual* update (United HealthCare, n.d.).

Technology assessments are advisory. They are but one input to United's coverage decisionmaking process. Although the Medical Policy Manager is responsible for incorporating a TA recommendation into coverage policy, the Medical Director drafts the technology assessment document. The format of the TA is such that it is easily converted to a policy-coverage statement.

Drugs are dealt with separately from procedures and devices. Diversified Pharmaceutical Services (DPS), which was a United specialty company, manages United's local health plans' pharmacy benefits. Although sold in 1994 to SmithKline, DPS is under contract with United to continue managing pharmacy benefits for another six years.

Clinical practice guidelines, of which about 20 are developed by United each year, may result from one of two sources: a national guideline or an internal practice guideline.

A national guideline, either from AHCPR or from a medical-specialty society, may provide the basis for the development of a United practice guideline. The sources of information it uses are verified, and the document is converted to United's guideline format. The guideline is then reviewed by United corporate medical directors, medical directors of selected health plans, and United's Chief Medical Officer. A guideline is sometimes reviewed by non-United physicians expert in the area.

Internal practice guidelines are developed similarly to technology assessments. Guidelines, following the specified organizational review process, are distributed in the quarterly update of the *Medical Management Manual* (United HealthCare, n.d.).

University HealthSystem Consortium[8]

The University HealthSystem Consortium (UHC), an association of 70 academic health centers (AHCs), was formed in 1984 by 23 university hospitals. Its mission is "to maintain and strengthen the competitive position of its individual members and their network partners in their respective health care markets" (University Hospital Consortium, 1994). UHC's initial focus was to obtain group-purchasing economies for its members. Today, it is organized around the following activities: group purchasing of major capital acquisitions, pharmaceuticals, intravenous (IV)–delivery products, materials and supplies; information resource services; value management; and market management.

Under *value management*, the Clinical Practice Advancement Center (CPAC) of UHC has programs related to clinical information management; clinical process improvement and measurement (benchmarking, guidelines use, and outcomes management); clinical research; and technology assessment. CPAC, formerly called the Technology Advancement Center (TAC), was created in 1988 to provide UHC members with an expert resource in "technology development, assessment, acquisition and management" (University Hospital Consortium, 1994). This statement reflects the complex and multifaceted orientation of hospitals toward medical technology.

Market management focuses on helping UHC members to analyze changes in local health markets and formulate appropriate strategic responses for managing enrolled populations, to obtain national contracts for UHC members' managed care products, to analyze capitation arrangements, to design primary-care networks for contracting in an increasingly capitated-plan market, and to guide specialty-care contracting. A central element in this area is the UHC market evolution model, which evaluates the implications for an AHC of local-market penetration by managed care plans.

Technology assessment at UHC began in 1989 with a member committee–directed effort. In 1991, UHC concluded that more structure was needed and assigned a staff member to the TA effort.

---

[8]In October 1995, UHC formally changed its name from University Hospital Consortium to University HealthSystem Consortium.

Currently, six FTEs are devoted to TA; outside consultants are used as needed.

The effort today is directed to "evaluating and comparing the safety, effectiveness, efficiency, appropriateness, cost and clinical outcomes of new and existing technology and disseminating the critical information provided by such assessments" (Matuszewski, 1995). *Technology assessment* has been defined by the principal UHC staff officer as "the process that examines the available evidence to form a conclusion as to the merits or role of a particular technology in relation to its possible use, purchase, or reimbursement in current medical practice" (Matuszewski, 1995).

Priorities for TA are established by a staff review of the literature and an annual survey of UHC members. The annual surveys have generated a steadily increasing number of distinct topics: about 100 in 1992, about 150 in 1993, and 199 in 1994. A technology is considered for assessment if it is used with a large number of patients; is controversial, expensive, risky, or unproven; has reimbursement difficulties; has multiple accepted treatment uses or diagnostic methods; or displays unexplained variation in medical practice or outcomes. The TA program issues approximately 10–12 TAs per year, with an additional 18–20 new-drug monographs. These assessments list appropriate uses, promising but unproven uses, and inappropriate uses of a given technology. UHC also publishes *Technology Assessment Monitor*, a guide to the published TAs of other organizations; and a monthly newsletter, *Technology Alert*.

In short, UHC has developed a TA effort that is embedded in an integrated program of related activities and responds to the needs of its members for information on the use of high-impact medical technologies. It does so by literature review, consensus panels, surveys of member practices, analyses of UHC databases, benchmarking of best practices, giving feedback to its members through its reports, and, most recently, through reports and focused educational conferences on members' uses of best-practice information. UHC TA documents are available for purchase for $50–$100 to any interested party. In addition, under a contractual arrangement with the Department of Veterans Affairs, all DVA member hospitals now receive UHC TA products.

THE NEW ORGANIZATIONAL PATTERN OF TA

In the past decade, a strong, decentralized TA capability has developed in the private health care sector of the United States, consisting of a small number of national organizations and a growing number of larger health plans. In this context, the federal government is only one player in a decentralized TA community, and one whose volume of output and product timeliness is modest. Moreover, the federal government is in a relatively weak position to exert leadership within this TA community along the lines envisaged for it in the 1970s and 1980s.

The decentralized organization of private-sector TA has developed along the following lines.

First, two organizations—Blue Cross Blue Shield Association and ECRI—have experienced strong growth in response to increased private-sector demand. Now conducting approximately 40 TAs a year, BCBSA has expanded its assessments beyond a service to its member plans and now offers a subscription service to all entities who will pay. Building from its base of hospital-oriented device evaluation, ECRI has also developed a subscription service, whereby subscribers can request TAs on specific medical devices, pharmaceuticals, and clinical procedures, in addition to obtaining assessments on topics done for several parties.

Second, several organizations have confronted or are confronting complicated organizational challenges. The American College of Physicians, whose Clinical Efficacy Assessment Program has long made it a leader in performing quality assessments, has been financed over time by a combination of contracts, foundation grants, internal ACP funds, and volunteer time. Whether this resource base will be adequate to sustain the CEAP in the next decade remains to be seen. The American Medical Association DATTA program, after a contraction due to budgetary cuts several years ago, appears to have stabilized its level of effort, has augmented its consensus-based activity with more-systematic reviews of the literature, and has developed a subscriber base. The American Hospital Association technology program, which also contracted earlier in this decade following changes in the organization's leadership and a subsequent review of all AHA services, also appears to have stabilized as a member-service effort, including the distribution of assessments of the University Hospital Consortium.

Third, constituency TA organizations have emerged in the past decade that serve *special clientele* or provide differentiated products. The University HealthSystem Consortium, for example, has probably served its members best by its aggressive efforts to analyze the implications of mainly managed-care-driven changes in the medical marketplace for academic health centers. In addition, however, UHC has developed, as part of a multifaceted clinical-practice-improvement effort, a TA program that responds to the needs of its 70 university hospital/health system members. Given its technical competence and its demand-driven program, UHC may emerge in the next decade as a strong national organization that can address the TA needs of the hospital sector, especially as hospitals evolve into integrated health delivery systems. In the past year, UHC's arrangements with both the American Hospital Association and the Department of Veterans Affairs for the distribution of its TA documents suggest this possibility.

TEMINEX, another constituency organization, was developed to serve the TA needs of The HMO Group, an organization of 30 group- and staff-model health maintenance organizations. Finally, in Minnesota, the Institute for Clinical Systems Integration (ICSI), which was created in response to an RFP from the Business Health Care Action Group, serves the needs of about 20 Minnesota health plans not only for clinical guidelines but also for TA.

Some TA organizations can be defined in terms of *differentiated products* rather than specific clientele. HAYES, for example, has chosen to produce a large number of TA reports very rapidly and to update them on a regular basis. Its assessments do not involve the staff input of a BCBSA or an ECRI, but it appears now that they do respond to a market need.

Fourth, several national insurance and managed care organizations, such as Prudential, Aetna, and United HealthCare, have developed substantial internal staff capabilities for conducting technology assessments, as well as for monitoring the TAs of others for a market of their local health plans. As a way to make or guide coverage decisionmaking for their member health plans, these organizations are reviewing the scientific literature more systematically than before. They are also creating evaluative capabilities relating to clinical practice guidelines and health services research.

Fifth, several individual health plans have well-developed TA capabilities. Group Health Cooperative of Puget Sound, for example, has had long-standing internal committees for evaluating new technologies (procedures and devices) and pharmaceuticals, and for developing prevention guidelines and therapeutic and diagnostic practice guidelines. Within the past two years, Group Health has begun to link these related efforts, all of which share a common methodology, into an integrated system—a system that is also supported by an internal physician-education effort focused on evidence-based medicine and by a high-quality health services research unit. Overall, the organization is making substantial data-system investments. Harvard Community Health Plan also has a TA effort as a part of its overall quality-improvement efforts. Kaiser-Permanente of Southern California is developing an integrated approach, within a new department, to practice guidelines and technology assessment.

At the beginning of this chapter, we described the organization of contemporary technology assessment in the United States as "highly decentralized." This is clearly the case. But the pluralistic pattern of *centralization and decentralization*, which is not easy to describe, has at least the following characteristics:

- *Centralized TA* under the aegis of the federal government, or under a private nonprofit entity, has not emerged.

- *Distributed centralization* has emerged within TA. The federal government is but one player and has a much more limited role than it envisioned a decade ago. This role is now shared with several private organizations, such as BCBSA, ECRI, HAYES, and University HealthSystem Consortium, which generate assessments for national markets.

- *Dedicated centralization* is also apparent, in which national organizations such as TEMINEX, Aetna, Prudential, and United HealthCare perform TAs for their own organizational members or affiliates.

- *Regional decentralization*—in which organizations such as the Institute for Clinical Systems Integration, Group Health Cooperative of Puget Sound, and Harvard Community Health Plan produce assessments for their own organizations, usually linking clinical practice guidelines and TA—has also been observed.

Coordination of TA activity in the above context is based on the flow of information among decentralized institutions, not on top-down administrative processes. The *producers/sellers* of TAs are quite aware of their competitors' products, assessment agendas, and customer base. The *buyers* of TAs are similarly aware of the range of available TA products and obtain assessments from multiple sources, often routinely. Information flows easily in this complex organizational environment.

In short, a robust analytical capability for technology assessment currently exists in the private sector of health care. Issues of content—the analytical and methodological strategies that characterize private-sector TA—are examined systematically in the next chapter.

REFERENCES

Catalona, W.J., Smith, D.S., Ratliff, T.L., Dobbs, K.M., Coplen, D.E., and Yuan, J.J., 1991. "Measurement of prostate specific antigen in serum as a screening test for prostate cancer," *New England Journal of Medicine*, Vol. 324, p. 1156ff.

Chalmers, T.C., 1994. "Implications of meta-analysis: need for a new generation of randomized control trials," in McCormick, K.A., Moore, S.R., and Siegel, R.A., eds., 1994. *Clinical Practice Guidelines Development: Methodology Perspectives*, Washington, DC, Agency for Health Care Policy and Research (AHCPR Publ. No. 95-0009), Department of Health and Human Services.

ECRI, 1995. *1995 Catalog*, Plymouth Meeting, PA.

Eddy, D.M., ed., 1991. *Common Screening Tests*, Philadelphia, PA, American College of Physicians.

Group Health Cooperative of Puget Sound, 1995. *Guidelines: Prostate Specific Antigen (PSA) As a Screening Test for Prostate Cancer*, Seattle, WA, GHCPS.

Handley, M.R., Stuart, M.E., and Kirz, H.L., 1994. "An evidence-based approach to evaluating and improving clinical practice: implementing practice guidlines," *HMO Practice*, Vol. 8, No. 2 (June), pp. 75–83.

Handley, M.R., and Stuart, M.E., 1994. "The use of prostate specific antigen for prostate cancer screening: a managed care perspective," *The Journal of Urology*, Vol. 152 (November), pp. 1689–1692.

Institute for Clinical Systems Integration (ICSI), 1995. *Objectives and Operating Structure*, Minneapolis, MN.

Institute of Medicine (IOM—Goodman, C., ed.), 1988. *Medical Technology Assessment Directory*, Washington, DC, National Academy Press.

Institute of Medicine (IOM—Mosteller, F., ed.), 1985. *Assessing Medical Technologies*, Washington, DC, National Academy Press.

Matuszewski, K.A., 1995. "Technology assessment," in Oleske, D.M., ed., *Epidemiology and the Delivery of Health Care Services: Methods and Applications*, New York, Plenum Press, pp. 123–148.

Sox, H.C., ed., 1987, 1990. *Common Diagnostic Tests: Use and Interpretation*, 1st ed., 2nd ed., Philadelphia, PA, American College of Physicians.

Stecher, T.J., Evans, R.W., Mosser, G., Reed, M.K., and Smith, J.C., 1995. "Technology assessment at the Institute for Clinical Systems Integration and Health Partners," *HMO Practice*, Vol. 9, No. 1 (March), pp. 22–26.

Stuart, M.E., Handley, M.A., Thompson, R.S., Conger, M., Timlin, D., 1992. "Clinical practice and new technology: prostate specific antigen (PSA)," *HMO Practice*, Vol. 6, No. 4, pp. 5–11.

Taubes, G., 1996. "Looking for the evidence in medicine," *Science*, Vol. 272 (April 5), pp. 22–24.

TEMINEX Report: Study #26, September 1994. *Intravenous Immunoglobulin for the Prevention of Recurrent Infections in Pediatric Patients*, Buffalo, NY, The HMO Group.

United HealthCare, n.d. *Medical Management Manual*, Buffalo, NY.

University Hospital Consortium, 1994. *The University Hospital Consortium: An Overview*, Oak Brook, IL.

Weiner, J.P., and deLissovoy, G., 1993. "Razing a Tower of Babel: a taxonomy for managed care and health insurance plans," *Journal of Health Politics, Policy, and Law*, Vol. 18, No. 1 (Spring), pp. 75–101.

Chapter Three

THE CONTENT OF TECHNOLOGY ASSESSMENT

In this chapter, we consider the *content*—the analytical and methodological strategies—of TA. These strategies include the emergence of a sharp focus on evidence-based assessments and the implications of that focus for consensus-based decisions; the evaluation of the financial implications of medical technologies, with special attention to cost-effectiveness analysis; the expansion of the scope of TA to include the evaluation of drugs *after* FDA approval for marketing; settled issues, such as organizational decisions supported by TA, evaluative criteria, priority-setting, and stage of technology development; and open issues, such as the relation of TA to clinical trials and to medical information systems.

THE EVALUATIVE CONTEXT OF TA

The past decade has seen the quiet but forceful emergence of health services research as a major factor in the formulation of U.S. health policy and in the delivery of health services. Although technology assessment is an integral part of health services research, it has had a complicated relationship to that endeavor that now is being clarified. We discuss this contextual issue here.

TA in medicine received strong impetus from both the creation of the Office of Technology Assessment in 1972 and the establishment of a health program within OTA soon thereafter. Although never more than a modest source of support for external investigators, OTA was instrumental in initiating the legislation that created the National Center for Health Care Technology (NCHCT) in 1978, an agency that was initially given administrative status within the Public Health

Service (PHS) parallel to that of the National Center for Health Services Research (NCHSR). Although NCHCT was conceived of as a TA-related *research* organization, it received an administrative delegation of authority from the Surgeon General *to advise Medicare on coverage decisions*. When NCHCT ended in 1982, it was absorbed into NCHSR as a subordinate Office of Health Technology Assessment (OHTA). Its residual, quasi-regulatory, Medicare TA advisory functions were retained, but it basically lost its research sponsorship role. This subordination of technology assessment to NCHSR, and later to its successor organization, the Agency for Health Care Policy and Research (AHCPR), continues to the present.

With a greater concern for delivery of health services and the measurement of quality than for technology assessment, health services research has had a different organizational identity, and has lacked the controversial responsibility of advising Medicare on coverage decisions. In the past decade, it has seen the emergence of research on effectiveness, outcomes, and appropriateness:

- **Effectiveness:** *Effectiveness*, what works in day-to-day clinical practice, differs from *efficacy*, what works under carefully controlled conditions, such as a randomized clinical trial. The concept of effectiveness provides the intellectual basis for going beyond the narrower FDA determination of efficacy for drugs and devices and also provides the basis for evaluating claims about procedures. It focuses on how diagnostic and therapeutic interventions contribute to patient outcomes. An "effectiveness" initiative sponsored by the Health Care Financing Administration in 1988–1989, for example, set the stage for the creation of a Medical Effectiveness Program within AHCPR in 1989 (Roper et al., 1988; IOM, 1989; IOM—Heithoff and Lohr, 1990).

- **Outcomes:** *Outcomes* are primarily the benefits to patients of clinical intervention for a given disease state or illness. The focus on medical outcomes reflects, among other things, a several-decade-long evolution of the conceptual approach to quality measurement (Donabedian, 1966) from concern for *structural measures* of quality (e.g., nurse/patient ratios) to *process measures* (e.g., adherence to diagnostic and therapeutic regimes believed to influence patient outcomes) to a more recent concern for *outcomes* (IOM—Lohr, 1990). This outcomes focus has also expanded the range of outcomes that should be measured, from mortality and from clinical and laboratory values of health to include the functional, health status, and health-related quality of life (Stewart and Ware, 1992; Patrick and Erickson, 1993).[1]

• **Appropriateness:** *Appropriateness* means that the benefits of in tervention exceed the risks when clinicians use effective medical procedures for given patients presenting with specific character- istics (Brook et al., 1986). Not all effective procedures are appro- priate for all patients. Thus, clinical judgment by a physician is necessary to relate population-based data on effectiveness and outcomes to specific patients and their circumstances.

The past decade has also witnessed the development of clinical prac- tice guidelines. *Guidelines* attempt to synthesize and codify the sci- entific evidence in the clinical literature about the effectiveness of medical interventions. Guidelines have a long history in medicine, but received a major impetus in the 1989 legislation that established AHCPR (Eddy, 1996). That agency's development of guidelines has resulted in, among other things, increased rigor in evaluating the scientific underpinnings of clinical practice (IOM—Field and Lohr, 1990, 1991). Although intended as guides to physician behavior, not as rules to override physician discretion in specific cases, guidelines *are* intended to be used in operational settings.

Substantial commonality in methods notwithstanding, a certain amount of confusion attends the relationship between TAs and guidelines. Some argue that "clinical practice guidelines can be viewed as a unique form of technology assessment that is intended to affect clinical decisions directly, as well as indirectly, through in- surance payment or other policies that are linked to those guide- lines" (OTA, 1994). Advocates of this view see TA as the umbrella un- der which other guidelines are developed. As a practical matter, however, many guidelines are generated without reference to TA and many guideline developers are either unaware of or agnostic about the relationship with TA. At best, these developers regard TA as but one element in a set of evaluative activities.

-----

[1]The relative importance of process and outcome measures is anything but settled. See, for example, Brook, McGlynn, and Cleary, 1996.

Although it is possible to develop a coherent statement of the conceptual relationship between TA and guidelines, it may be impossible to generate one that commands widespread agreement. Moreover, it may be that the issue is getting sorted out in a practical way in operational settings. That said, Table 3.1 presents dimensions for differentiating between TAs and guidelines that suggest that TAs and guidelines have in common a philosophy of *evidence-based evaluation* of medical interventions: Both may be oriented to a *specific technology or procedure;* if not, it is because guidelines are often directed to the management of a *clinical condition or disease entity,* sometimes with respect to a defined patient population. In this regard, guidelines are likely to assess a family of technologies, whereas the focus of a TA is usually on a specific technology, i.e., a drug, device, or procedure. TAs and guidelines also are likely to support different organizational decisions: TA is linked strongly to coverage decisionmaking, whereas guidelines are linked to clinical practice. TAs and guidelines share a concern for *existing* technologies, but *new* technologies are basically the province of TA. This focus on new technologies means that data for TA tend to be scarcer than for guidelines.

Clearly, these two activities have much in common and, depending on how they are defined, may also have distinct characteristics of their own. In the operational settings described in the preceding chapter, two patterns are apparent in the relationship between TA and guidelines. First, those organizations that have few direct relationships with physicians *do* conduct technology assessments; typically, they *do not* develop clinical practice guidelines. Analytic organizations such as BCBSA and ECRI, membership organizations such as UHC, and the corporate offices of managed care organizations having many health plans display this pattern. Second, those organizations that have direct working relations with physicians, such as local HMOs, are moving increasingly both to conduct TAs *and* to develop practice guidelines.

Given the above definitions and distinctions, we can now look specifically at the various aspects of the content of technology assessment.

Table 3.1

Technology Assessment and Clinical Practice Guidelines

Dimension of Comparison	Technology Assessment	Clinical Practice Guidelines
Subject of assessment	Specific medical technology or procedure	• Specific technology • Family of technologies to manage a clinical condition or disease entity • Clinical condition or disease entity
Assessment questions	Clinical safety, efficacy, effectiveness, and health outcomes; cost-effectiveness	Clinical effectiveness, appropriateness, and outcomes
Stage of development of assessed technology	New and existing	Existing
Organizational decision supported	Coverage and reimbursement, procurement of equipment, management of technology costs	Clinical practice and patient management; patient information
Philosophy and methods	Evidence-based	Evidence-based
Data availability	Limited	Ranges from limited to extensive

ANALYTICAL AND METHODOLOGICAL STRATEGIES

Evidence-Based Technology Assessment

In general, technology assessment has been concerned with second-order consequences of technology: the social, economic, legal, and ethical effects and implications of technology for society. By contrast, the central questions of TA in medicine focus more on the evaluation of immediate (first-order) clinical issues:

• Is a given technology or procedure safe?

• Is it efficacious under conditions of rigorous control?

• Is it effective under conditions of normal clinical use?

- What is its clinical effectiveness relative to alternative technologies?

- Is it cost-effective relative to other technologies?

However, the broader social, legal, and ethical implications of medical technology may receive special attention, frequently by bioethicists. A good example of this phenomenon is the Program of Ethical, Legal, and Social Implications (ELSI) of the Human Genome Project.

An underlying philosophic change in the orientation to TA became evident in interviews conducted for this research, clearly indicating that a major semantic shift had occurred between the mid-1980s and the mid-1990s in the way TA is described. In interview after interview, both face-to-face and on the telephone, regardless of geographic location or institutional affiliation, the recurring refrain was "We have an *evidence-based* [TA] assessment procedure." In fact, both TA and clinical practice guidelines are increasingly described as evidence-based.

The consistency with which the *evidence-based* terminology is used from one organization to another is remarkable in itself and, it is safe to say, reflects conscious value and policy choices by the individuals and organizations using the term. One source of this semantic and philosophic shift is the work centered at the Department of Clinical Epidemiology and Biostatistics of McMaster University (Evidence-Based Medicine Working Group, 1992). McMaster University's Evidence-Based Medicine Working Group, which includes individuals from other Canadian and U.S. institutions, has generated a series of papers in the *Journal of the American Medical Association* under the heading of "Users' guides to the medical literature" (Guyatt and Rennie, 1993; Oxman et al., 1994; Guyatt et al., 1993, 1994; Jaeschke et al., 1994a, b; Levine et al., 1994; Laupacis et al., 1994; Richardson et al., 1995a, b). The conceptual core of this literature is this: "Evidence-based medicine *de-emphasizes* intuition, unsystematic clinical experience, and pathophysiologic rationale as sufficient grounds for clinical decision making and *stresses the examination of evidence from clinical research*" [emphasis added] (Evidence-Based Medicine Working Group, 1992).

In this country, David Eddy has contributed strongly to the shift in thinking with his contrast of physicians' traditional, implicit approach to the evaluation of health practices with an approach characterized by the "explicit and systematic analysis of evidence, estimation of outcomes, calculation of costs, and assessment of preferences" (Eddy, 1992, 1996). In fact, the increasing rigor and clinical focus of much of health services research and the diffusion of such research into clinical use contributes to this general development of evidence-based medicine. Evidence of the penetration of this thinking into clinical practice is found in Stuart and Handley's manual, *An Evidence-Based Approach to Changing Clinical Practice* (n.d.), which is used as the basis for physician education within Group Health Cooperative of Puget Sound.

Ideally, comprehensive assessments of a medical technology or procedure include evaluating the relationship of a given intervention to the scientific evidence about effectiveness, to the health outcomes of patients, to costs, and to patient preferences. Such assessments are motivated by a desire to reduce the variation in clinical practice that is unexplained by disease incidence, patient characteristics, or resources; to reduce or eliminate inappropriate use of medical procedures; and to promote the use of effective interventions. They are also intended to maximize the value of delivered services (either by maximizing outcomes for a given level of resources or minimizing resource use for a given level of health outcomes) through a process that relates the marginal cost of an intervention to its marginal benefit.

In this context, evidence-based assessments may include some or all of the following elements:

- Adoption of formal, explicit, and systematic methods of evaluation of the evidence and the rejection as inadequate of methods that are informal, implicit, and unsystematic (e.g., reliance upon informal consensus of experts)

- Systematic review of the published (and sometimes unpublished) clinical literature

- Combining of the results of multiple studies by meta-analysis

- Extraction and presentation of evidence from the literature in evidence tables that are related to specific clinical questions (see below)

- Grading of the quality of the literature from which the data are drawn

- Compilation of a balance sheet that arrays the benefits and harms of a given clinical intervention

- Formulation of a recommendation regarding coverage, clinical practice, or the need for additional clinical evaluation in relation to (1) what is known, (2) what is not known and about which no conclusion can be drawn, and (3) what is not known but about which expert clinical opinion (consensus) exists.

We present two examples of evidence tables here (see also Guyatt et al., 1995). The first example is from the educational manual developed by Michael Stuart and Matthew Handley of Group Health Cooperative of Puget Sound for instructing physicians about evidence-based clinical practice. Table 3.2 is the tool for evaluating the quality of the evidence in a study. The highest grade (Grade 1, in this example) is given for randomized controlled trials; the lowest grade (Grade 5) is given for "expert opinion" (Stuart and Handley, n.d., p. 25). Table 3.3 shows the use of this tool for a Grade 1 study of the active management of labor in childbirth. This table is one of several used in a decision-analytic illustration of guideline development; it is presented here only to indicate how evidence is displayed, not to discuss this particular guideline.

The second example of evidence tables is from a study sponsored by the American College of Physicians on the clinical efficacy of magnetic resonance imaging for neuroimaging (Kent et al., 1994) reported in the scientific literature. The data for these tables were drawn from a literature review that identified 3,125 citations in the peer-reviewed medical literature from 1987 through November 1993. After reviews, technical reports, case reports, and other publications describing fewer than 30 original-case patients had been screened out, 285 papers remained for further review. Of these, 156 papers were selected for review for diagnostic accuracy or diagnostic impact, therapeutic impact, or patient outcomes. The following tables indicate how the quality of these papers was graded:

- Table 3.4 indicates the bases for classifying studies of a diagnostic test with respect to the question: "Are the study

Table 3.2

Tool for Evaluating the Quality of Evidence in a Study (see Table 3.3)

Study Evaluation Tool

Reference _____

What is the Grade of the Evidence?
◊   Grade 1
-    Randomized controlled trials.

◊   Grade 2
-    Non- randomized prospective cohort studies.

◊   Grade 3
-    Non-randomized historical cohort studies.
-    Other studies using non-experimental designs (e.g., population-based studies, case control studies) with meticulous attention to study execution. Such studies will have utilized some or all of the following:
  -    careful measurement of controls to decrease confounding errors
  -    adequate sample size

◊   Grade 4
-    Case series

◊   Grade 5
-    Expert opinion

Size of the study? n = _____

How valid is the study?
- If the study used a randomized design, were patients properly randomized? (Treatment and control groups are similar in all important variables)
- Were all patients accounted for at the end of the study? (Patients may be lost because of treatment affects or adverse outcomes)
- Was the study population relevant? (Does the study population represent the population you are interested in?)
- Were relevant outcomes measured and were they measured blindly? (Intermediate vs. clinically significant outcomes)
- What was the length of follow up?
- What was the effect of the intervention? (What was the reported difference between treatment and control groups, e.g., RR, ARR, OR?)
- What is the likelihood that the findings were from chance? (What were the p value, confidence interval?)
- Were adverse outcomes of the intervention reported?

What were the conclusions?
- Does the data presented support the conclusions reached by the authors? (To what extent did the authors extrapolate their findings to reach their conclusions?)

SOURCE: Stuart, M.E., and Handley, M.A., n.d. *An Evidence-Based Approach to Changing Clinical Practice*, Seattle, WA, Group Health Cooperative of Puget Sound, p. 25. Reprinted with permission.

Table 3.3

Evidence Table: Active Management of Labor

Study	Study Size & Characteristics	Labor & Delivery Outcomes				Infant Outcomes
			Control Group	Treatment Group	Adjusted OR	
Lopez-Zeno et al. NEJM. 1992;326:450–454. *A controlled trial of a program for the active management of labor.* Chicago, IL	Randomized once labor diagnosed N = 705 315 in treatment group 354 in control group	C section rate	14.1%	10.5%	* (0.36–0.95)	No significant differences in: • birth weight • 5-minute Apgar • umbilical artery pH • NICU admit • seizures • deaths • days in hospital • meconium • delivery for FHR abnormalities • transfusion • shoulder dystocia
		Operative vaginal delivery rate	33%	28%	NS	
		Duration of labor (hr)	8.15 ±2.75	6.45 ±2.75	p < 0.0001	
		% not delivered after 12 hrs.	18.9%	4.6%	p < 0.001	
		% receiving oxytocin	66.1%	71.2%	N/S	
		% requiring oxytocin decreased or stopped	57.5%	46.4%	p < 0.05	
		Chorioamnionitis	9.9%	4.6%	p < 0.01	

*Adjusted for maternal age, height, weight gain, gestation age, birth weight, epidural, cervix on admission, payer. Reduction not significant (P = 0.18) when not adjusted.

Comments

• Study size not sufficient to evaluate fetal outcomes adequately (beta error possible).
• Rate of epidural (~70%) very high in both groups.
• Historical control C section rate 22.4% nullips suggests Hawthorne effect. C-section rate reported for women meeting AML criteria. Treatment group includes 6 women randomized to AML but protocol not followed.

SOURCE: Stuart, M.E., and Handley, M.A., n.d. *An Evidence-Based Approach to Changing Clinical Practice*, Seattle, WA, Group Health Cooperative of Puget Sound, p. 60. Reprinted with permission.

Table 3.4

Three Dimensions to Classification of Studies of a Diagnostic Test*

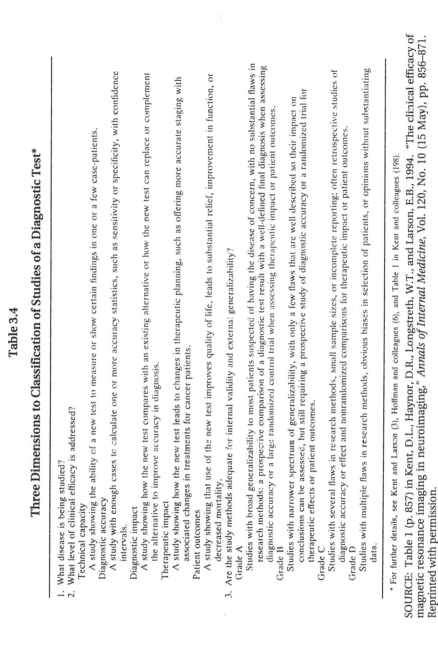

1. What disease is being studied?
2. What level of clinical efficacy is addressed?

   Technical capacity

   A study showing the ability of a new test to measure or show certain findings in one or a few case-patients.

   Diagnostic accuracy

   A study with enough cases to calculate one or more accuracy statistics, such as sensitivity or specificity, with confidence intervals.

   Diagnostic impact

   A study showing how the new test compares with an existing alternative or how the new test can replace or complement the alternative to improve accuracy in diagnosis.

   Therapeutic impact

   A study showing how the new test leads to changes in therapeutic planning, such as offering more accurate staging with associated changes in treatments for cancer patients.

   Patient outcomes

   A study showing that use of the new test improves quality of life, leads to substantial relief, improvement in function, or decreased mortality.

3. Are the study methods adequate for internal validity and external generalizability?

   Grade A

   Studies with broad generalizability to most patients suspected of having the disease of concern, with no substantial flaws in research methods: a prospective comparison of a diagnostic test result with a well-defined final diagnosis when assessing diagnostic accuracy or a large randomized control trial when assessing therapeutic impact or patient outcomes.

   Grade B

   Studies with narrower spectrum of generalizability, with only a few flaws that are well described so their impact on conclusions can be assessed, but still requiring a prospective study of diagnostic accuracy or a randomized trial for therapeutic effects or patient outcomes.

   Grade C

   Studies with several flaws in research methods, small sample sizes, or incomplete reporting; often retrospective studies of diagnostic accuracy or effect and nonrandomized comparisons for therapeutic impact or patient outcomes.

   Grade D

   Studies with multiple flaws in research methods, obvious biases in selection of patients, or opinions without substantiating data.

* For further details, see Kent and Larson (3), Hoffman and colleagues (6), and Table 1 in Kent and colleagues (198).

SOURCE: Table 1 (p. 857) in Kent, D.L., Haynor, D.R., Longstreth, W.T., and Larson, E.B., 1994. "The clinical efficacy of magnetic resonance imaging in neuroimaging," *Annals of Internal Medicine*, Vol. 120, No. 10 (15 May), pp. 856–871. Reprinted with permission.

methods adequate for internal validity and external general-izability?" (Kent et al., 1994, p. 857).

- Table 3.5 lists and grades the studies indicating therapeutic impact or changes in patient outcomes, with a footnote explaining the method grade (Kent et al., 1994, p. 858).

- Table 3.6 presents the evidence table grading studies of diagnostic accuracy for various conditions. (Additional tables present information on diagnostic accuracy for carotid artery disease, multiple sclerosis and related syndromes, and imaging in the spine.) Grading was based on the following criteria (Kent, et al., 1994, p. 859): A—"if the study had more than 35 patients with and more than 35 without the pathologic abnormality in question, drawn from a clinically relevant sample whose clinical symptoms were completely described, whose diagnoses were defined by an appropriate reference standard, and whose magnetic resonance images were technically of high quality and were evaluated independently of the reference diagnosis." D—"if they had no credible reference standard for diagnosis, or if the test result and determination of final diagnosis were not independent, or if the sample size was smaller than 35 for patients with and without the disease, or if the source of the patient cohort could not be determined or was obviously influenced by the test results (work-up bias)."

Kent et al. (1994, p. 856) summarize the grading of the evidence in the following way: "Of 3,125 citations retrieved, 156 studies with original data could be rated according to methodologic criteria for study design. One article contributed grade A quality information about diagnostic accuracy, 28 were grade B or C, and 113 were graded D. One randomized trial and 2 comparison studies con-tributed grade B or C information about the impact on therapeutic choices. Only 2 studies surveyed health status before and after mag-netic resonance scanning."

What are the implications of evidence-based technology assessments for consensus processes? First, as the above discussion indicates, the literature on evidence-based methodology is substantial and increas-ing, reflecting the growing importance attached to systematic review of the literature and, simultaneously, a turning away from *unsystematic expert opinion* as a means for assessing the scientific bases of medicine.

Second, although the 1985 IOM report (IOM—Mosteller) included a section on "group judgment processes" in its lengthy chapter on TA methodologies, concern for such processes is seldom expressed today.

Third, an evidence-based TA done to determine clinical effectiveness often becomes one *input,* among several, to a coverage and reimbursement decision. In such cases, decisions about the use of a technology or procedure often require that financial, legal, and other factors be considered, and that competing values be weighed. Some collective or consensual decision process is likely to be used in the weighing.

Fourth, there are indications that such consensus processes are becoming more systematic in response to the evidence-based movement. On the one hand, for example, the DATTA program of the American Medical Association has evolved in recent years from basically an opinion poll of expert physicians, without reference to the literature, to a poll in which respondents are now provided a literature review at the same time that they are asked for their expert opinions on a procedure. On the other hand, the consensus-development program of the National Institutes of Health has always conducted extensive literature searches in support of its efforts, although it has not systematically compiled evidence tables or graded the quality of the literature in its supporting reviews.

Fifth, when terminally ill patients wish access to procedures that are regarded by advocates as the "best available" and by skeptics as "experimental" and on which the evidence about the effectiveness is lacking or ambiguous, health plans often invoke some expert-consensus process in reaching their decision on specific cases. The process may involve blending evidence-based information with expert judgment about the particular circumstances of the case and the appropriateness of the treatment for the given patient.

In summary, the dominant theme encountered in the course of this research was the search for evidence-based assessments of technologies. Clearly, less reliance is being placed on the ability of individual clinicians to synthesize the scientific literature, integrate that

Table 3.5

Studies Indicating Therapeutic Impact or Changes in Patient Outcomes*

Study (Reference)	Methods	Types of MRI Scan	Conclusion	Method Grade†
Ten-Haken et al. (120)	Prospective comparison of radiation treatment volumes based on CT or MRI, using composite as reference standard (n = 15)	0.35 T, 0.5 T, 1.5 T	MRI defined larger volumes closer to standard. Interobserver variation was of similar magnitude, so one cannot conclude that MRI is better for treatment plans.	C
Simon (83)	Observations of 210 patients having CT or MRI for dementia in community practices; prospective controlled study	Not stated	Counts of treatment changes and outcomes: observed 26 diagnosis changes leading to 4 treatment changes with no improvements.	D
Szczepura et al. (218)	Prospective comparison of pre-MRI treatment plans with post-MRI plans in 782 consecutive patients, who also were surveyed before and after for disability and distress	1.5T	Major change in diagnosis in 13% of patients. Treatment plans changed in 27%, including abandonment of 8% of planned operations. Disability and distress were worse 6 months after scans because of underlying disease severity.	D
Dixon et al. (213)	Prospective prescan, postscan survey for various diagnoses (n = 200)	Not stated	22% of actual physician plans were changed by MRI.	D
Teasdale et al. (216)	Randomized controlled trial of CT or MRI as first imaging test for posterior fossa (n = 1020)	0.15 T, posterior fossa coils	CT was ordered after MRI in 6% of patients. MRI was ordered after CT in 19% of patients. MRI changed 6% of treatment plans. CT changed 2% of treatment plans.	B

Table 3.5—continued

Study (Reference)	Methods	Types of MRI Scan	Conclusion	Method Grade†
Sze et al. (119)	Review of contribution of MRI or CT to treatment plans in patients having both tests for brain tumors (n = 75)	1.5 T, 5 mm	In 68 patients, there were no discordant images. Among 7 patients with imaging disagreements, treatment was based on CT in 3 patients and on MRI in 4 other patients.	C
Franken et al. (217)	Treatment plans recorded before and after MRI scans for various diagnoses (n = 189)	0.5 T	Referring doctors thought 16% of diagnoses were changed and an unspecified number of treatments also changed. No rating of appropriateness of changes and no outcomes.	D
Shuman et al. (116)	Pre-MRI radiation treatment plans for tumors compared with post-MRI plans (n = 30)	0.15 T	Reviewers independent of treatment planners found 53% of plans showed measurable change in treatment field after MRI. No comparison with CT-based treatment plans was done.	D

* Definitions of terms discussed in text and references (see Kent and Larson [3]). CT = computed tomography; MRI = magnetic resonance imaging. T = tesla.
† Grade A studies are large-scale randomized trials, whereas grade B studies are small randomized trials. Grade C requires some concurrent comparison of MRI to an alternative. Grade D studies were prospective surveys of treatment plans.

SOURCE: Table 2 (p. 858) in Kent, D.L., Haynor, D.R., Longstreth, W.T., and Larson, E.B., 1994. "The clinical efficacy of magnetic resonance imaging in neuroimaging," *Annals of Internal Medicine*, Vol. 120, No. 10 (15 May), pp. 856–871. Reprinted with permission.

Table 3.6

Diagnostic Accuracy of Magnetic Resonance Imaging for Various Conditions

Study (Reference)	Participants in Study*	Type of MRI (Alternative)	Methods Quality Grade†	Magnetic Resonance or Alternative Technology		
				Sensitivity (95% CI)‡	Specificity (95% CI)‡	Comments
Buchfelder et al. (113)	Patients with definite pituitary Cushing disease; 141 patients from 1982 to 1991	1.5 T, 3 to 4 mm	C	0.61 (0.48 to 0.73)	1.0 (0.79 to 1.0)	MRI and CT not done on same patients
		(CT with contrast, 2-mm thin slices)		0.53 (0.43 to 0.63)	0.88 (0.64 to 0.99)	
Yetkin et al. (32)	Volunteers with no disease (n = 131), all adult ages, with or without hypertension	1.5 T, 5 mm	B	. . .	0.66 (0.57 to 0.74)	Image positive if unexplained focal hyperintensities in white matter were seen
Golomb et al. (78)	Older volunteers who were normal on several cognitive tests and had no hypertension or other medical problems (n = 154)	1.5 T, 6 mm	B	. . .	0.67 (0.58 to 0.74)	Image positive if any hippocampal atrophy was seen (half of abnormal persons had unilateral atrophy)
Erkinjuntti et al. (77)	Patients with dementia (n = 34); controls (n = 39)	1.5 T, 5 mm	B	0.59 (0.41 to 0.75)	0.96 (0.93 to 0.99)	Positive image was atrophy of entorhinal cortex

Table 3.6—continued

Study (Reference)	Participants in Study[*]	Type of MRI (Alternative)	Methods Quality Grade[†]	Magnetic Resonance or Alternative Technology		
				Sensitivity (95% CI)[‡]	Specificity (95% CI)[‡]	Comments
Adler et al. (223)	Patients with hemifacial spasm (n = 37); controls (n = 16)	1.5 T, MRA	B	0.65 (0.47 to 0.80)	1.0 (0.79 to 1.0)	Positive image was vessel compression of ipsilateral brainstem
Orrison et al. (29)	Unselected, consecutive series (n = 126); clinical and surgical outcomes determined by careful follow-up	1.5 T	C	0.96§ (0.87 to 0.995)	0.50§ (0.26 to 0.74)	Positive images of cranial pathology from readings kept independent from final clinical and surgical diagnoses
		0.064 T		0.96§ (0.89 to 0.99)	0.70§ (NA)	
		(Contrast CT)		0.94§ (0.84 to 0.98)	0.68§ (NA)	
Kawamoto et al. (28)	Hypertensive and normal patients age >60 with no symptoms or history (n = 88)	0.6 T, 10 mm	B		0.86 (0.76 to 0.94) 0.58 (0.47 to 0.68)	Image positive if scan had >4 lacunae

Table 3.6—continued

Study (Reference)	Participants in Study[*]	Type of MRI (Alternative)	Methods Quality Grade[†]	Magnetic Resonance or Alternative Technology		
				Sensitivity (95% CI)[‡]	Specificity (95% CI)[‡]	Comments
Jackson et al. (128)	Temporal lobe pathologic abnormality in patients having epilepsy surgery (*n* = 81)	0.3 T, 9 mm	C	0.93 (0.76 to 0.99)	0.86 (0.57 to 0.98)	Image positive if hippocampal sclerosis was seen
Fazekas (30)	Volunteers normal by history and physical examination (*n* = 87)	1.5 T	C	...	0.55 (0.44 to 0.66)	

* Numbers in parentheses are number of patients contributing to accuracy data. Actual statistics in some articles are based on the number of organs imaged, such as two carotid arteries per patient or several disk levels per patient. CT = computed tomography; MRI = magnetic resonance imaging; NA = not available; T = tesla.
† Methods quality grades described in text.
‡ Confidence intervals are from tables in reference 237.
§ Sensitivity and specificity from the points closest to the upper left of the receiver-operating characteristic curve in article.

SOURCE: Table 3 (p. 859) in Kent, D.L., Haynor, D.R., Longstreth, W.T., and Larson, E.B., 1994. "The clinical efficacy of magnetic resonance imaging in neuroimaging," *Annals of Internal Medicine*, Vol. 120, No. 10 (15 May), pp. 856–871. Reprinted with permission.

synthesis into their working clinical knowledge, and modify their practice in response. Reliance is increasingly placed on more-scientific evaluations of the evidence in the clinical literature.

TA and Economic Analysis

There is an extensive health policy literature on cost-effectiveness. A recent book edited by Sloan (1995), for example, includes more than 20 pages of references. It discusses the evaluation of clinical effectiveness, the estimation of health effects as quality-adjusted life-years (QALYs), which go beyond expected survival and also estimate quality-of-life improvements, the measurement of costs, the analysis of incremental cost-effectiveness, the monetary valuation of health benefits, discounting, statistical issues, decision trees and Markov models, and the use of cost-effectiveness analysis in actual decisionmaking. The technology assessment literature has included conceptual and case-study applications of cost-effectiveness analysis at least since the early 1980s (OTA, 1980; Warner and Luce, 1982).

Historically, the practical emphasis of TA has been on clinical effectiveness, not on cost-effectiveness. It remains there today, given that so much of medicine lacks clear scientific evidence of effectiveness. By contrast, the use of cost-effectiveness analysis in TA has been relatively limited, for two reasons: First, until recently, the marketplace *incentives* to use such analysis have not been strong enough to encourage its development as a practical decisionmaking tool. Second, the *methodologies of practical application*, as distinct from methodologies of research, have not been well developed.

Both the incentives to use cost-effectiveness analysis (CEA) and the methodologies of application are changing. Driven by cost-containment and quality-assurance objectives, health plans are increasingly examining the clinical effectiveness of interventions *and* their financial implications. Attention to these financial implications reflects the increasingly held belief among many health-plan managers that technology affects the costs of the plan more strongly than it affects revenues. Consequently, cost-effectiveness becomes more important as a management tool.

The initial steps to link TA and the cost effects of technology typically involve using TAs as inputs to financial decisions to estimate, for example, the effect of a technology on the premium or cost structure of the health plan or on its revenue-generating potential in a local health market. This practice foreshadows the formal inclusion of cost-effectiveness analysis in TA.

We observed two patterns among the organizations interviewed in this research: an arm's-length separation between TAs focused on clinical effectiveness and health-plan decisions about the cost effects of a technology or procedure, and a single body responsible for assessing both clinical effectiveness and cost-effectiveness.

When an "arm's-length" relationship is established between a technology assessment and decisions about financial implications, an evidence-based review of the literature conducted for and reviewed by an expert panel restricts itself to a recommendation about clinical effectiveness. This TA recommendation is then sent to another body, such as a benefits committee, whose responsibilities include making financial decisions for the plan. This two-step process separates the conduct of an assessment from the decision about its use. It is favored by many and deemed essential by some, the reasoning being that only an arm's-length relationship ensures that financial considerations do not distort the scientific assessment of clinical effectiveness.

In Minnesota, for example, the Institute for Clinical Systems Integration develops practice guidelines and TAs for HealthPartners, an HMO, and other participating medical groups. ICSI restricts itself to assessing the science, i.e., to assessing the clinical effectiveness. HealthPartners then uses these assessments as inputs to policy decisions in which financial considerations are a major, if not dominant, element. ECRI, to take another example, markets its TAs partly on the basis of their independence from the economic implications of health-plan coverage and payment decisions.

In the second pattern, the body conducting a TA is responsible for decisions about both the clinical effectiveness and the financial implications of a technology. One example is the Pharmacy and Therapeutics (P&T) Committee of Group Health Cooperative of Puget Sound, which assesses the clinical effectiveness of a new drug in relation to that of existing drugs in the same class, then estimates the economic effect on the plan, taking into account the price of the new drug, its probable use, substitution effects for other medications, etc. If the estimated additional costs to GHC are less than $50,000 per year, the committee acts for GHC; if the estimated costs are greater than $50,000, the P&T recommendation goes to the Executive Council for a decision about adding the new drug to the formulary. The Committee on Medically Emerging Technologies of GHC has similar authority.

Neither of these patterns involves the use of formal CEA. There are signs, however, that TA performers are moving toward incorporating cost-effectiveness analysis into technology assessments. BCBSA has taken the initial steps to include cost-effectiveness analysis in its TAs of diagnostic procedures. In mid-1995, it conducted a clinical assessment of positron emission tomography myocardial perfusion imaging (PET MPI) for the detection of coronary artery disease (CAD). It focused on indications for "intermediate-risk" patients (defined as having a probability of between 25 and 75 percent of having CAD). PET was compared with four alternative *noninvasive* diagnostic technologies—(1) planar scanning (PLANAR), using thallium-201 or technitium 99m sestamibi scintography; (2) single-photon emission computed tomography (SPECT), using thallium-201 or technitium 99m sestamibi; (3) exercise echocardiography (ECHO); and (4) exercise electrocardiography (ETT, or treadmill testing)—and with *invasive* coronary angiography. The health outcomes that were evaluated include the mortality and morbidity of the noninvasive tests, the mortality and morbidity of coronary angiography, and the mortality and morbidity associated with CAD and any of its treatments, relative to four test results (true positive, false positive, true negative, false negative).

The clinical literature provided no direct evidence that PET imaging for the detection of CAD had an effect on health outcomes. The search for evidence, therefore, focused on comparisons of test performance and on how each of the four possible test results might influence subsequent patient management and health outcomes. The two assessment questions were

*   For detection of CAD in people at intermediate risk, what were the probabilities of the four outcomes for PET? What were the probabilities of each of these outcomes for the other noninvasive tests for CAD?

- If PET and alternative noninvasive tests were used to determine which patients should receive coronary angiography, how did the test performance characteristics influence the outcomes of CAD?

To be included in the assessment, published papers had to indicate that angiography and at least one of the noninvasive tests were performed on the same patients, that sufficient data on the noninvasive tests were available so that the results of coronary angiography could be predicted precisely for the four outcomes, and that an FDA-approved PET radiotracer was used for the PET studies. Studies had to be of high quality, the study populations had to be individuals at intermediate risk, i.e., the same as the patients of concern to the assessment, and additional inclusion and exclusion criteria were applied.

The results of the clinical TA for test performance were that PET scanning was shown to be "at least as accurate" as alternative noninvasive tests for CAD in those at intermediate risk of the disease. PET was more sensitive than all the other tests, and it was at least as specific as all the other tests, save echocardiography, which is less sensitive. For the effect on patient management and health outcomes, PET yielded minimal gains in QALYs when compared with SPECT, the next most costly noninvasive test.

A companion cost-effectiveness analysis was conducted for this clinical assessment of PET MPI by Dr. Alan Garber, a member of the BCBSA Medical Advisory Panel, and Dr. Neil Solomon (BCBSA, 1995). The analysis adopted a societal (or national) perspective, which includes all social costs and benefits regardless of their distribution. It sought to determine a cost-effectiveness ratio, or the "dollar cost per unit improvement in health" of PET MPI when compared with the five alternatives. The study focused on the differences in costs between the intervention and its alternatives, and in health effects, which were estimated as QALYs. The study discounted future costs and health effects at an annual rate of 2 percent. Cost data were obtained from physician-fee surveys, a large insurer, a large HMO, and the literature.

The CEA showed that PET costs per procedure were much higher than SPECT ($1,500 versus $470 Medicare reimbursement). PET resulted in slightly more QALYs than SPECT, but slightly fewer than avoiding noninvasive tests entirely and going directly to coronary angiography. And the cost-effectiveness ratio, or the dollar cost of an additional QALY, was on the order of $0.5 million when PET was compared with SPECT. When the level of CAD prevalence was varied for 55-year-old men (25 percent, 50 percent, and 75 percent), immediate angiography was slightly better than PET for all three levels, at slightly lower cost.

The study summarized the lessons of the cost-effectiveness analysis in this way (BCBSA, 1995):

- The computational challenge is increased by the number of alternative diagnostic technologies and the treatments considered.

- Relevant data are sometimes difficult to obtain and, therefore, some assumptions are necessarily arbitrary.

- Assumptions regarding patient management after diagnosis are also required.

- Simplification of the analysis is possible, but how to simplify it is not always obvious.

- Sensitivity analyses to compensate for uncertainty are complex when the number of uncertain parameters is large.

- Criteria for identifying the intermediate-risk patient are critical, but how to apply them is not straightforward.

- Results of diagnostic tests may be operator-dependent.

Even so, Garber and Solomon conclude, CEA generates useful but unexpected results: "In any complex question (and especially in evaluations of diagnostic tests), the apparently simple rapidly becomes complex. Data limitations become a prominent problem. Also it is somewhat difficult to locate facts by literature search even when data on a particular question exist. For example, relevant data may be reported in papers that are mainly addressed to a different topic" (BCBSA, 1995).

Thus, the feasibility of CEA, performed by a skilled analyst, as a complement to the assessment of clinical effectiveness, was demonstrated. The analysis also provided substantial insight beyond that of a clinical-effectiveness assessment and identified some of the challenges of application.

For new-drug evaluation, CEA is being used increasingly by pharmaceutical companies seeking to demonstrate the cost-effectiveness of their products when compared with alternative drugs. This is true both in the United States and in Canada (Detsky, 1993). Hillman and colleagues, in 1991, reported that they had conducted 33 economic analyses for 15 pharmaceutical companies since 1978 (Hillman et al., 1991). Such analyses, they indicated, were increasingly being used for marketing purposes and to obtain formulary approval.

In the past few years, the discussion of including CEA in the evaluation of drugs has turned on the principles that ought to govern the reporting in the literature of cost-effectiveness analyses sponsored by drug firms (Hillman et al., 1991; Task Force on Principles for Economic Analysis of Health Care Technology, 1995), focusing on the minimization and control of bias. In this context, the editors of the *New England Journal of Medicine* issued a policy in 1994 regarding cost-effectiveness analyses that stipulated highly restrictive conditions for submitted papers to be considered for publication: Support from an industrial firm had to be to a nonprofit entity, not to an individual or group of individuals; written assurance of the authors' independence in all aspects of the study, analysis, and reporting of results was required; and the manuscript had to include all data, all assumptions on which data were based, and a description of any model used in the analysis (Kassirer and Angel, 1994). Quite clearly, the assessment of drugs by CEA has crossed an analytic threshold, and a controversy about reporting results has begun that is likely to continue for several years.

The wider use of CEA may be diffusing to the medical device industry. In 1995, a two-volume report was issued by Medical Alley of Minnesota: *Measuring Cost Effectiveness: A Roadmap to Health Care Value, Vol. 1: Issues and Methods, Vol. 2: A Technical Guide.* The report resulted from a task force that met "to produce a clear, concise publication that will provide any healthcare organization—no matter what their level of sophistication in presenting the value they add to healthcare—with a practical guide that will allow it to more effectively meet the needs of the current and future healthcare environment" (letter from Thomas L. Meskan, President, Medical

Alley, August 2, 1995). The mission of the task force was to state "a consensus position" describing cost-effectiveness analysis and to develop "a practical set of guidelines" to demonstrate or assess cost-effectiveness.

The Medical Alley task force developed a checklist of 12 items for assessing the value of a drug, device, procedure, use of knowledge, and/or process applied to human health. These items are indicated in Table 3.7.

The task force took a different conceptual approach to the economists' argument for a societal perspective on costs and benefits. It encouraged the "consideration of a community perspective" as part of a CEA, identifying this perspective as that of "the insurer,

Table 3.7

Medical Alley: Checklist for Addressing a Technology's Value

Foundations of Cost-Effectiveness Evaluation
1. Describe the technology and its potential benefits. Include demographic information and information on appropriate use.
2. State the perspective used to compare costs and benefits.
3. State which technology alternatives are compared.
4. State which analytic tools were used, and explain why they were chosen.

Measuring Costs
5. Describe the data sources used for all financial costs included in the evaluation.
6. State whether costs relating to productivity or lost work days (indirect costs) are included and listed separately.
7. Where appropriate, break down cost information into a per-member per-month rate for a given population.

Measuring Outcomes
8. Describe the dimensions of health outcomes included in the evaluation.
9. Describe the sources used to gather health outcomes data.

Issue of Time and Uncertainty
10. State the time horizon used to determine costs and outcomes.
11. Describe the discount rate(s) included in the analysis.
12. Test key assumptions using sensitivity analysis.

SOURCE: Medical Alley, 1995a. *Measuring Cost-Effectiveness: A Roadmap to Health Care Value. Vol. 1. Issues and Methods*, Minneapolis, MN, p. 8. Reprinted with permission.

the manufacturer, the clinic or hospital, the patient, or the entire population." It justified its community perspective as follows (Medical Alley, 1995a):

> A broad perspective, including the needs of an entire community, should be one of the considerations when conducting a cost effectiveness evaluation. A community perspective is more focused than a societal perspective, and allows for local decisions to be made concerning healthcare interventions. The Task Force defines community as the population receiving care from a health system. Membership may consist of individuals living within a geographic service area or persons in other well-defined sub-populations (e.g., those enrolled in a public or private health plan).

The basic issue in the debate between the societal and community perspectives is that the distribution of health risks, benefits, and costs may vary in ways that affect the results of the analysis. An example can clarify the distinction between societal and community perspectives. If a "well-defined sub-population" is compared with the national population, and the former is healthier for the clinical condition of interest (i.e., has a lower incidence of the condition), a given intervention whose per-treatment (unit) costs are the same in both settings would, by definition, be less costly in population (per capita) terms, and analysis would show the treatment to be more "cost-effective" in the sub-population. If, in addition, treatment outcomes of the patients drawn from the healthier sub-population were better than those in the national population, a cost-effectiveness analysis would favor the intervention in the community setting even more. This example leaves unaddressed what analysis of the costs and effects of the intervention in the community setting might show, addressing only the effect of adopting the community perspective: The analysis would not reveal the implications of the intervention in societal terms. The tension between the society and the community perspectives, which is simultaneously an analytic, economic, and political issue, must be negotiated in both political and economic terms if CEA is to become integral to technology assessment.

Research-based advocates of CEA are unlikely to see the Medical Alley report, because it is priced very high ($125) and is not easily accessible to those accustomed to following the journal literature.

Those who do may be inclined to dismiss the report as elementary: Both volumes are relatively slim, neither provides many illustrative cases, and the technical guide adds relatively little to the volume on issues and methods. But dismissal of the report would be unfortunate. A more useful response would be to view it as the basis for a sustained discussion between TA analysts and the medical device industry about the problems of CEA application, because real-world application of CEA is the market test that this method must meet in the years ahead, not whether economists are persuaded of its utility.

After the Medical Alley report was completed, *Cost-Effectiveness in Health and Medicine* (Gold et al., 1996) was published. The work of an expert panel convened by the U.S. Public Health Service, this book will undoubtedly be the benchmark for cost-effectiveness analysis in health services research for some time to come. Whether the incentives of the health care marketplace will result in the adoption of CEA as a tool for practical decisionmaking, however, is the question that advocates of this technique now face.

The Broadened Scope of TA: Drug Evaluations

Although the OTA definition of *medical technology* encompasses "drugs, devices, and medical and surgical procedures used in medical care, and the organizational and supportive systems within which such care is provided," TA has generally been restricted to medical *devices* and medical and surgical *procedures*. The assessment of *drugs* has been left to the Food and Drug Administration and to reliance on its premarket review process. However, in recent years, the scope of TA has been broadened to include the evaluation of drugs *after* FDA approval for marketing.

The FDA premarket evaluation and approval of a drug, on the basis of evidence from two adequate and well-controlled clinical studies of its safety and effectiveness, has, under fee-for-service medicine, been a fixed referent for payers, insurers, and managed care organizations. FDA approval used to result in a near-automatic decision by these parties to include a medication in a formulary or in a benefit package.

However, the evaluation of prescription drugs is changing in complex ways.

Fast-Track Reviews. First, FDA remains under constant pressure to reduce the time for review of a New Drug Application (NDA). One consequence of this pressure is that FDA has introduced *accelerated approval* of new drugs in the areas of oncology, HIV and AIDS, and other life-threatening illnesses, a process known as "fast-track" review. A familiar feature of fast-track review is the use of surrogate end points, or proxies for clinical end points or outcomes, which are measured by laboratory values but lack supporting clinical outcomes data. An example is the use of CD-4 counts[2] as a measure of efficacy of drugs to treat AIDS, as distinct from clinical measures of effectiveness. Although accelerated approval speeds new drugs to market, it does not generate the clinical outcome measures valued by insurers and managed care organizations, thus weakening the basis of these organizations' reliance on FDA decisions.

More-Complex Clinical Trials. Second, drug firms—on their own initiative but in response to increased competitive forces in the marketplace—have increased the complexity of clinical trials in two ways. They have begun to use *cost-effectiveness analysis* in their evaluation of new drugs, both in analyzing competing product-development investment alternatives and, by integrating CEA into clinical trials, in generating results that are used in marketing new drugs (as being more "cost-effective" than their competitors). Drug firms have also increasingly used *quality-of-life measures* in clinical trials for new drugs, thus expanding the relevant health outcomes beyond mortality, morbidity, laboratory, and clinical measures, to include measures of how well patients function and perceive the quality of their lives. The use of quality-of-life measures reflects the fact that the most effective differentiation of the effects of a new drug, especially in the treatment of chronic disease, is often measured in quality-of-life terms. These two developments put more drug-effectiveness information into play, but from the sponsors of the drugs themselves.

Pharmacy and Therapeutics Committees. Independent of these changes in drug evaluation, a change in the competitive health marketplace has occurred that is very important from a TA per-

---

[2]The number of CD-4 cells in a blood sample is a measure of immune-system strength. Generally, the CD-4 count decreases as HIV progresses.

spective.   Under pressures of cost containment, an increasing proportion of *drug-prescribing decisions* have shifted from the individual physician's office-based practice to health plan and hospital-based pharmacy and therapeutics committees.   These committees decide which drugs to list in their formulary.   (The United States has been characterized as the last major industrialized country of the world to move from the individual physician to a corporate entity as the principal customer of prescription drugs.)

Although these P&T committees have existed in hospitals and HMOs for some time, they once were made up mainly of pharmacists.   Now, they have a more diverse membership that reflects drug prescribers and users within the health plan.   P&T committees constitute an infrastructure that is being reinvigorated to scrutinize more closely than before the addition of new drugs to the formulary.   Of analytical interest to P&T committees are the clinical effectiveness of a new drug, especially in relation to other drugs having similar therapeutic capabilities, and the cost of the new drug relative to that of existing drugs.   These committees take the safety and effectiveness requirements of the FDA as a starting point, but go beyond FDA judgments to make their own determinations about clinical effectiveness.

Two distinct institutional patterns for the evaluation of new drugs are apparent from the organizations we researched.   In some organizations, such as the BCBSA Technology Evaluation Program, a single committee considers all new technologies (drugs, devices, procedures).   This "full-service" approach also characterizes UHC, for example, and is the direction in which ECRI is moving.   More frequently, however, as in the case of Group Health Cooperative of Puget Sound, a P&T committee will deal with questions related to new drugs, but a new-technologies committee will deal with medical devices and procedures.   However, these two patterns are not fixed and may very well change over time.

Off-Label Uses of Approved Drugs. Off-label uses of FDA-approved drugs and biologics pose difficult TA challenges.   Although FDA approves a specific drug for a particular clinical indication, a physician may prescribe any FDA-approved drug for any indication.   This practice is widespread in oncology: There are so few effective drugs that a compound approved for use against a particular tumor will quickly be used experimentally against many other tumors.   The TA challenges raised by off-label uses stem from the absence of scientific evidence of clinical effectiveness for the particular indication and from the demand for use of any medication that offers some hope for terminal patients.

Off-label uses receive a good deal of TA attention. For example, BCBSA, at its June 1995 meeting, considered the following off-label uses of FDA approved drugs: epoetin alfa therapy for myelodysplastic syndromes (to stimulate the increase of hemoglobin for transfusion-dependent patients) and for chronic anemia of cancer; human antihemophiliac factor maintenance therapy for severe hemophilia A; intravenous immunoglobulin for refractory systemic lupus erythematosus; epoetin alfa therapy following allogeneic bone marrow transplantation or high-dose chemotherapy with autologous stem-cell support; interferon therapy for off-label oncology indications for lymphomas, leukemias, or plasma-cell malignancies and, separately, for solid tumors; and serum tumor markers for the diagnosis and monitoring of breast cancer.

A different off-label issue was considered by Blue Shield of California, at the March 22, 1995, meeting of its Medical Policy Committee on Quality and Technology. The committee reviewed the use of prolotherapy for the treatment of chronic back pain. Prolotherapy consists of a series of intraligamentous injections in the spine, using a solution of dextrose, glycerin, and phenol—all of which are FDA-approved medications, but not approved in solution form for treatment of chronic back pain. The Medical Director of Blue Shield of California, using the BCBSA criteria, concluded that clinical studies conducted since Blue Shield's policy on prolotherapy was adopted in 1992 did not permit conclusions about the effect of prolotherapy on health outcomes; that a judgment about whether the treatment improved net health outcomes could not be reached; and that the criteria that prolotherapy be as effective as established alternatives and that improvement be attainable outside investigational settings were not applicable. After discussion, the committee voted that prolotherapy "remains investigational."

To take another example of assessments of off-label uses of FDA-approved drugs, in June 1995 the Blue Shield of California committee considered indications for the use of intravenous immunoglobulin (IVIG) for a variety of conditions. FDA had approved IVIG for the following five indications: (1) treatment of primary immunodeficient states; (2) prevention of bacterial infections in patients with hypogammaglobulinemia and/or recurrent bacterial infections associated with B-cell chronic lymphocytic leukemia (CLL); (3) prevention and/or control of bleeding in a patient with idiopathic thrombocytopenic purpura (ITP); (4) prevention of infection in HIV-infected children; and (5) prevention of infection and/or graft-versus-host disease in bone-marrow-transplant patients. Prior Blue Shield reviews of IVIG indications in October 1990 and October 1992 had resulted in decisions to cover all but the fourth item in the above list, as well as neonates disposed to Group B streptococcal infections, Kawasaki disease, coagulopathy due to inhibitors of antihemophiliac factor (Factor VIII), and Guillain-Barré syndrome. Based on the Medical Director's 1995 review of the literature and resulting recommendation, the committee added chronic inflammatory demyelinating polyneuropathy (CIDP), pediatric HIV disease, and refractory dermatomyositis to the list of "eligible for coverage" indications. But the other proposed IVIG uses were not supported by "well-designed clinical trials published in the peer-reviewed literature," and as a result all other indications were deemed "investigational."

Settled Issues

At the same time that many issues are complicating TA, as well as broadening it, several issues in technology assessment appear to have been settled in the past decade: the organizational decisions supported by TA, the evaluative criteria for assessing a technology, setting priorities for conducting assessments, and the stage of technology (new, established, obsolete) that is the object of TA.

Organizational Decisions. Coverage and reimbursement decisions are the principal decisions of insurers and health plans that are supported by TA, especially TA focused on new technologies. A recurring question of TA is, Do the data provide a sufficient basis for determining that a given technology or procedure satisfies a set of criteria that make it "eligible for coverage," i.e., eligible for inclusion in the set of covered benefits? Coverage decisions may arise when a new technology or procedure for which a general medical policy has yet to be established is diffusing into clinical practice. They sometimes arise when a plan must make a specific decision about the immediate treatment of a particular patient; i.e., a physician has a patient for whom a given procedure is being considered and inquires about the clinical effectiveness of the procedure.

In addition, TAs are increasingly being used in support of clinical practice guidelines. However, this practice varies as a function of whether the organization has a mandate to go beyond TA advice on coverage decisions. National organizations, such as BCBSA and ECRI, which have no organizational or legal relationship to physicians' practice of medicine, do not prepare clinical practice guidelines. Managed care organizations such as Harvard-Pilgrim HealthCare, HealthPartners, or Group Health Cooperative, which do have working relationships with their affiliated physicians, engage in the development of practice guidelines.

Evaluation Criteria. Technologies and procedures that are selected for assessment need to be evaluated by certain criteria. The most clearly developed and widely cited criteria for evaluating medical technologies have been developed by the Blue Cross Blue Shield Association. These five criteria, cited in Chapter Two (Table 2.1) in a more elaborate form, can be abbreviated as follows:

1. The technology must have final approval from the appropriate government regulatory bodies.
2. The scientific evidence must permit conclusions concerning the effect of the technology on health outcomes.
3. The technology must improve the net health outcome.
4. The technology must be as beneficial as any established alternative.
5. The improvement must be attainable outside the investigational settings.

Organizations that conduct TAs typically use some variant of these criteria. Organizations also may vary how explicitly and formally the criteria are incorporated into their decision processes.

Priority-Setting. How to set priorities is one methdological issue that has received a good deal of attention for determining which technologies to assess. This issue arises because the number of candidates for assessment is always substantial, resources are always limited, and some selection of assessment topics must be made. Moreover, priority-setting by governmental agencies can affect the private interests of those advocating particular interventions, and thus is often a highly political process.

Priority-setting for TA was outlined in a 1992 IOM report (IOM—Donaldson, 1992) prepared for the AHCPR. The report proposed the following seven-step process: (1) select priority-setting criteria and assign a weight to each; (2) solicit nominations of candidates for technology assessment; (3) reduce a large list of nominees to those on which to obtain the data needed for priority-ranking; (4) obtain the needed data set; (5) for each topic, assign a score for each relevant attribute; (6) calculate priority scores for each topic and rank topics in order of priority; and (7) have an AHCPR panel review the priority list and select assessment topics. The proposed selection criteria focused on clinical conditions: prevalence, cost, clinical practice variations, burden of illness, likelihood that results of the assessment would affect patient outcomes and costs, and ethical, legal, and social issues. A similar report published in 1995 addressed priority-setting for clinical practice guidelines (IOM—Field, 1995). These reports define the idealized processes of priority-setting.

Organizations that conduct TAs often use these priority-setting models as a point of departure for designing their operational systems. Typically, their actual processes adapt the models to the practical realities they confront. BCBSA, for example, publishes a monthly list for its members and subscribers of assessments in progress, planned TAs, and topics under consideration. It determines its TA priorities by considering suggestions from both its member-subscribers and its professional staff. The staff monitor 25–30 journals and the trade press, and attend scientific meetings. In addition, BCBSA surveys its member-clients directly for their suggestions. Finally, the last agenda item of every Medical Advisory Panel meeting is a review of the priority list, which is updated continually.

ECRI priorities for technology assessment derive from the interaction between its professional staff and client-subscriber demands. This interaction, which occurs formally and informally on a sustained basis, is based on receiving many calls, daily for the past 20 years, on devices and device-using procedures. In addition, many technologies that receive an initial ECRI assessment become topics for continuing surveillance and, potentially, for reassessment. Reassessment priorities are set when the literature reports a change in the clinical status of a technology.

Priority-setting by the many TA organizations discussed in Chapter Two reveals some clustering around the "hot button" topics of the day. But priorities also reflect the particular needs of the different TA organizations and their clients. Thus, the number and range of TAs actually conducted are greater than could be expected from a single TA organization.

Stage of Technological Development. The literature often specifies the domain of TA as "new and emerging," "existing," and "obsolete-but-still-used" technologies. Those engaged in the conduct of TA on a regular basis, however, are mainly concerned with *new technologies*, which may mean the initial application of a technology or new uses of an existing technology, e.g., an off-label use of an FDA-approved pharmaceutical. Performers of TA often estimate that as much as two-thirds of their efforts is devoted to new technologies and one-third to existing technologies. Obsolete technologies do not occupy much attention, as a practical matter. However, the balance between the assessment of new and existing technologies is empirical, deriving more from practical needs than from policy, and is likely to fluctuate over time.

Open Issues

In the course of this study, those who responded to the interviews raised several TA-related issues that had not been anticipated in the early stages of the research. Here, we briefly discuss two of those issues—clinical trials and data systems—because both are important in the generation and evaluation of medical technology.

Clinical Trials. The relationship of technology assessment to clinical trials is complicated, and comes into play most directly for TAs focused on the evaluation of new medical technologies (drugs, devices, and medical and surgical procedures) for making coverage decisions.

In the main, responsible insurers, managed care plans, and integrated delivery systems wish to make coverage decisions about a technology's effectiveness on the basis of scientific data. For cost and clinical reasons, such organizations do not wish to finance ineffective treatment. To make informed coverage decisions about new clinical technologies and procedures, they need good-quality clinical data. So they depend on the clinical-trials literature for information about clinical effectiveness, especially for procedures that do not involve FDA-regulated trials done in support of drug or medical device evaluation.

The quality of the clinical-trials literature is not uniformly high, however. Thus, when TA organizations conduct evidence-based literature reviews to identify critical studies and to compile evidence tables, and when complementary efforts attempt to grade the key studies on the basis of methodological quality, their analysts often give relatively low grades—no better than a C, according to several respondents—to those studies. The most-frequent reasons for the low grades are the paucity of data on controls, or the lack of controls; lack of clarity in the definitions of patient groups and outcomes of interest (sample-selection criteria are not specified, or there are few controls for bias, or sample size is too small); objective measures of outcome have not been defined, and outcome data for baseline and post-intervention have not been obtained; the period of follow-up post-intervention is too short relative to the natural history of the disease; or follow-up reporting is incomplete.

Fortunately, one unintended consequence of the prevailing robust analytical TA and guidelines capability in the private health care sector has been the formation of a cadre of critics of the clinical-trials literature among the ranks of TA performers and guidelines developers. Unfortunately, a concomitant feedback loop has not been generated to enable the information about the critical appraisals of that literature to flow back to the sponsors or performers of such trials.

FDA regulatory requirements impose substantial rigor on drug trials, so this issue is more serious for procedures than for pharmaceutical firms' trials of new drugs. FDA controls include a detailed section of the *Code of Federal Regulations* (21 C.F.R., Subchapter D, "Drugs for human use," U.S. General Services Administration, 1991), a *Guideline for the Format and Content of the Clinical and Statistical Sections of New Drug Applications* (U.S. FDA, 1988), the review of NDAs by FDA professional staff, and the final review, by an external expert advisory committee, of an application, which contains the results of trial data.

For procedures that do not require FDA approval, however, sponsors and performers of clinical trials have practically no connection to those who eventually will evaluate and use the results of their work. One source of this problem, according to some managed care officials, is that the *management* of government-sponsored clinical trials is often weak: There are too many trials, of too weak design (often too few controls), with too slow a patient accrual rate, and trials are often conducted without reference to outcomes of interest to payers or patients. Issues of common design across a number of related trials have not been addressed with an eye to accumulating results through meta-analyses (Chalmers, 1994).

Another problem, the critics argue, is that trials are not always intended to establish clinical effectiveness, even though their basic rationale is that the accumulation of scientific results in laboratory and animal studies is sufficiently promising to warrant trials involving human subjects. Results are often not germane to the needs of those responsible for medical decisions about effective and appropriate interventions in the settings in which physicians normally encounter patients and for which insurers and managed care organizations must pay. One source of this difficulty, in the view of some respondents, is that trials are often driven by the norms and values of academic medicine, which include the quest for tenure, the creation of an academic niche in the medical marketplace, and the search for revenue for the institution.

Four related problems have been identified. The first is that basic data about government-sponsored clinical trials are not easily available. For example, many parties report frustration at being unable to obtain an inventory of government-sponsored clinical trials. Second, the reporting of clinical-trial results in the scientific journals has not yet been standardized, although movement in that direction has been reported (Rennie, 1995). Third, responsible managed care and provider organizations have no mechanism for routinely indicating to the federal government their priorities for clinical trials or for indicating the patient-related outcomes that should be considered.

The fourth problem is that, from the perspective of NIH and the medical research community, payment for clinical trials has become much more complicated in the past decade than it was previously. Insurers were once looked upon as a source of payment for such trials, but have basically withdrawn from subsidizing research on "experimental" procedures. However, some insurers that were once reluctant to pay for clinical-trials research have now begun to think that paying for investigational care for beneficiaries enrolled in a clinical trial is reasonable, if some of the management issues discussed above are remedied. The issue of payment for clinical trials remains unresolved. A sustained discussion involving all parties is clearly needed.

TA and Data Systems.   The definition of *medical technology* has always encompassed "the organizational and supportive" technologies of health care, which might also be called "efficiency" technologies: computer-based information systems, electronic patient records, and physician and nurse workstations. Although they have often been ignored in the TA literature, these efficiency technologies intersect with therapeutic and diagnostic technologies. They are taking on added importance in the present environment, particularly since cost control is seen as a way to free up resources that might be allocated to other purposes, including new therapeutic interventions. If efficiencies can be gained through investments in information systems, the ability of providers and health plans to maintain delivered quality at lower costs will be enhanced.

However, the path from investments in data systems to lower-cost quality health care has not been a straight one. Several years ago, health services *researchers* hoped that large administrative databases would provide useful information about the effectiveness of clinical interventions. That hope has waned, if not evaporated, as the limits of existing databases and the prohibitive costs required to bring those databases to an acceptable level of usefulness have become apparent. Nevertheless, the efficiency technologies are, today, the focus of very substantial investments by *managers* of health plans, and these investments may create a capacity in the future to acquire both financial and clinical data in a way that can support a large number of plan decisions and data users.

A major issue that is related to but distinct from TA, therefore, is the need for sustained attention to the design of information systems that permit financial and clinical information to be linked and that would enable prospective studies to compensate for the absence of literature-derived data.

CONCLUSIONS

What conclusions can be drawn from this chapter?

First, TA is clearly one of a family of evaluative activities that are diffusing steadily within health care organizations. Health services research has provided the foundation for most of these activities—effectiveness, appropriateness, and outcomes research; quality assessment, quality assurance, and continuous quality improvement; technology assessment; and clinical practice guidelines. The federal government has often been the sponsor of many of these endeavors. However, at the federal government level, commonalities among these distinct efforts have often been lost sight of, because conceptual distinctions among the efforts have often been reified and then enshrined in specific programs or organizations, which have acquired their own supporting constituencies.

In the private sector of health care—including managed care—technology assessment is sometimes independent of clinical practice guidelines and sometimes closely related to them. And both of these activities have various relationships to applied health-services research. As these evaluative efforts diffuse further in the next decade, public and private decisionmakers should make it their priority to strengthen the common foundations of TA, practice guidelines, and health services research, i.e., the concern for clinical effectiveness in day-to-day clinical settings.

Second, the strength of the orientation to evidence-based assessments that characterized practically all respondents is the most significant finding to emerge from this research. Rigorous evaluation of clinical effectiveness, based on a systematic review of scientific and clinical evidence, has become the norm among the TA organizations interviewed for this study. For TA, and for other efforts to evaluate medical effectiveness, a priority of public- and private-sector decisionmakers should be to broaden, deepen, and generally strengthen this commitment to evidence-based assessment of the scientific foundations of clinical interventions. One benefit of such a commitment will be to bring the appropriate role of expert consensus into clearer focus.

In this evidence-based context, it is worth noting that the philosophy, underlying assumptions, and methods of TA have been set forth clearly in the literature (IOM—Mosteller, 1985; Sox, 1990; Eddy, 1991, 1992; IOM—Donaldson, 1992; and IOM—Field, 1995). In 1985, *Assessing Medical Technologies* (IOM—Mosteller) devoted a lengthy chapter to the following TA methodologies: randomized controlled trials; evaluations of diagnostic techniques; case series; case studies; registries and databases; sample surveys; epidemiologic methods; surveillance methods; quantitative synthesis methods, primarily meta-analysis; group judgment methods; cost-effectiveness and cost-benefit analyses; mathematical modeling; and social and ethical issues in technology assessment.

The IOM—Mosteller report recommended that a greater commitment be made to generating primary data on the safety and efficacy of *new* medical and surgical procedures, to determining the cost-effectiveness and public-policy implications of those procedures, and to postmarketing surveillance of drugs and medical devices, as well as of medical technology *already in use*. It also recommended increased research to improve the various methods of TA, both by increasing the use of the stronger methods and by strengthening the weaker methods. Finally, it recommended that increased resources be allocated for training researchers in medical technology assessment, both for advancing the methodology and for applying those methods to the many unevaluated technologies.

Although the methods of TA are obviously good enough at this time for operational use, it would be worthwhile to review the progress made in the decade since the IOM—Mosteller report in order to determine whether additional research on assessment methodology is warranted, especially for use in applied settings.

Third, the use of cost-effectiveness analysis in the assessment of medical technologies should be given continuing attention and should emphasize the conceptual, methodological, and data challenges of application in operational settings. The issue of societal versus community perspective, for example, deserves thorough discussion, as do the incentives that govern the use of CEA. However, the primary audience for this discussion is neither health economists nor policy analysts, but current and prospective users of CEA.

Fourth, the scope of TA should be recognized as having become increasingly *full-service:* It includes drugs, medical devices, and clinical procedures. Prior reliance on FDA evaluations of the safety and effectiveness of new drugs is now augmented. In many cases, reviews by pharmacy and therapeutics committees take an FDA evaluation as the *starting point* for formulary decisions, not as an automatic basis for adding a drug to a formulary.

Fifth, the weaknesses of the clinical-trials literature that are revealed by evidence-based assessments should become the basis for creating systematic feedback to the sponsors and performers of such trials. The priorities of payers, insurers, and managed care organizations for clinical trials should be systematically ascertained and communicated to the appropriate federal government and private-sector sponsors of such trials. The feedback could be obtained and the priorities could be set at an annual meeting sponsored by AHCPR or NIH. The meeting could focus on determining the top three to five clinical trials that payers and/or insurers believed were needed, and on addressing methodological and management issues related to clinical trials. Such a conference could also be the vehicle for examining the difficult issue of who should pay for clinical trials and under what circumstances.

REFERENCES

Blue Cross Blue Shield Association (BCBSA) Medical Advisory Panel, 1995. *Positron Emission Tomography Myocardial Perfusion Imaging for the Detection of Coronary Artery Disease—Cost Effectiveness Analysis,* Chicago, IL, June 29–30.

Brook, R.H., Chassin, M.R., Fink, A., et al., 1986. "A method for the detailed assessment of the appropriateness of medical technologies," *International Journal of Technology Assessment in Health Care,* Vol. 2, No. 1, pp. 53–63.

Brook, R.H., McGlynn, E.A., and Cleary, P.D., 1996. "Quality of health care: Part 2: Measuring quality of care," *New England Journal of Medicine,* Vol. 335, pp. 966–970.

Chalmers, T.C., 1994. "Implications of meta-analysis: need for a new generation of randomized control trials," in McCormick, K.A., Moore, S.R., and Siegel, R.A., eds., 1994. *Clinical Practice Guidelines Development: Methodology Perspectives,* Washington, DC, Agency for Health Care Policy and Research (AHCPR Publ. No. 95-0009), Department of Health and Human Services.

Detsky, A., 1993. "Guidelines for economic analysis of pharmaceutical products: a draft document for Ontario and Canada," *PharmacoEconomics,* Vol. 3, pp. 354–361.

Donabedian, A., 1966. "Evaluating the quality of medical care." *Milbank Memorial Quarterly,* Vol. 44, pp. 166–203.

Eddy, D.M., ed., 1991. *Common Screening Tests,* Philadelphia, PA, American College of Physicians.

Eddy, D.M., 1992. *A Manual for Assessing Health Practices & Designing Practice Policies: The Explicit Approach,* Philadelphia, PA, American College of Physicians.

Eddy, D.M., 1996. *Clinical Decision Making: From Theory to Practice,* Sudbury, MA, Jones and Bartlett.

Evidence-Based Medicine Working Group, 1992. "Evidence-based medicine: a new approach to the teaching of medicine," *JAMA,* Vol. 268, pp. 2420–2425.

Gold, M.R., Siegel, J.E., Russell, L.B., and Weinstein, M.C., eds., 1996. *Cost-Effectiveness in Health and Medicine*, New York, Oxford University Press.

Guyatt, G.H., and Rennie, D., 1993. "Users' guides to the medical literature," *JAMA*, Vol. 270, pp. 2096–2097.

Guyatt, G.H., Sackett, D.L., Cook, D.J., for the Evidence-Based Medicine Working Group, 1993. "Users' guides to the medical literature: II. How to use an article about therapy or prevention. A. Are the results of the study valid?" *JAMA*, Vol. 270, pp. 2598–2601.

Guyatt, G.H., Sackett, D.L., Cook, D.J., for the Evidence-Based Medicine Working Group, 1994. "Users' guides to the medical literature: II. How to use an article about therapy or prevention. B. What were the results and will they help me in caring for my patients?" *JAMA*, Vol. 271, pp. 59–63.

Guyatt, G.H., Sackett, D.L., Sinclair, J.C., Hayward, R., Cook, D.J., Cook, R.J., 1995. "Users' guides to the medical literature: IX. A method for grading health care recommendations," *JAMA*, Vol. 274, pp. 1800–1804.

Hillman, A.L., Eisenberg, J.M., Pauly, M.V., Bloom, B.S., Glick, H., Kinosian, B., and Schwarz, J.S., 1991. "Avoding bias in the conduct and reporting of cost-effectiveness research sponsored by pharmaceutical companies," *New England Journal of Medicine*, Vol. 324, pp. 1362–1365.

Institute of Medicine, 1989. *Effectiveness Initiative: Setting Priorities for Clinical Conditions*, Washington, DC, National Academy Press.

Institute of Medicine (IOM—Donaldson, M., ed.), 1992. *Setting Priorities for Health Technology Assessment: A Model Process*, Washington, DC, National Academy Press.

Institute of Medicine (IOM—Field, M.J., ed.), 1995. *Setting Priorities for Clinical Practice Guidelines*, Washington, DC, National Academy Press.

Institute of Medicine (IOM—Field, M.J., and Lohr, K.N., eds.), 1990. *Clinical Practice Guidelines: Directions for a New Program*, Washington, DC, National Academy Press.

Institute of Medicine (IOM—Field, M.J., and Lohr, K.N., eds.), 1991. *Clinical Practice Guidelines: From Development to Use*, Washington, DC, National Academy Press.

Institute of Medicine (IOM—Goodman, C., ed.), 1988. *Medical Technology Assessment Directory*, Washington, DC, National Academy Press.

Institute of Medicine (IOM—Heithoff, K.A., and Lohr, K.N., eds.), 1990. *Effectiveness and Outcomes in Health Care*, Washington, DC, National Academy Press.

Institute of Medicine (IOM—Lohr, K.N., ed.), 1990. *Medicare: A Strategy for Quality Assurance, 2 Vols.*, Washington, DC, National Academy Press.

Institute of Medicine (IOM—Mosteller, F., ed.), 1985. *Assessing Medical Technologies*, Washington, DC, National Academy Press.

Jaeschke, R., Guyatt, G.H., Sackett, D.L., for the Evidence-Based Medicine Working Group, 1994a. "Users' guides to the medical literature: III. How to use an article about a diagnostic test. A. Are the results of the study valid?" *JAMA*, Vol. 271, pp. 389–391.

Jaeschke, R., Guyatt, G.H., Sackett, D.L., for the Evidence-Based Medicine Working Group, 1994b. "Users' guides to the medical literature: III. How to use an article about a diagnostic test. B. What are the results and will they help me in caring for my patients?" *JAMA*, Vol. 271, pp. 703–707.

Kassirer, J.P., and Angel, M., 1994. "The journal's policy on cost-effectiveness analysis," *New England Journal of Medicine*, Vol. 331, pp. 669–670.

Kent, D.L., Haynor, D.R., Longstreth, W.T., and Larson, E.B., 1994. "The clinical efficacy of magnetic resonance imaging in neuroimaging," *Annals of Internal Medicine*, Vol. 120, No. 10 (May 15), pp. 856–871.

Laupacis, A., Wells, G., Richardson, W.S., Tugwell, P., for the Evidence-Based Medicine Working Group, 1994. "Users' guides to the medical literature: V. How to use an article about prognosis," *JAMA*, Vol. 272, pp. 234–237.

Levine, M., Walter, S., Lee, H., Haines, T., Holbrook, A., Moyer, V., for the Evidence-Based Medicine Working Group, 1994. "Users' guides to the medical literature: IV. How to use an article about harm," *JAMA*, Vol. 271, pp. 1615–1619.

McPherson, K., Wennberg, J.E., and Hovind, O.B., et al., 1982. "Small-area variation in the use of common surgical procedures: an international comparison of New England, England, and Norway," *New England Journal of Medicine*, Vol. 307, pp. 1310–1314.

Medical Alley, 1995a. *Measuring Cost Effectiveness: A Roadmap to Health Care Value, Vol. 1: Issues and Methods*, Minneapolis, MN.

Medical Alley, 1995b. *Measuring Cost Effectiveness: A Roadmap to Health Care Value, Vol. 2: A Technical Guide*, Minneapolis, MN.

Office of Technology Assessment (OTA), U.S. Congress, 1980. *The Implications of Cost-Effectiveness Analysis of Medical Technology*, Washington, DC, U.S. Government Printing Office.

Office of Technology Assessment, U.S. Congress, 1994. *Identifying Health Technologies That Work: Searching for Evidence*, Washington, DC, U.S. Government Printing Office.

Oxman, A.D., Cook, D.J., Guyatt, G.H., for the Evidence-Based Medicine Working Group, 1994. "Users' guides to the medical literature: VI. How to use an overview," *JAMA*, Vol. 272, pp. 1367–1371.

Oxman, A.D., Sackett, D.L., Guyatt, G.H., for the Evidence-Based Medicine Working Group, 1993. "Users' guides to the medical literature: I. How to get started," *JAMA*, Vol. 270, pp. 2093–2095.

Patrick, D.L., and Erickson, P., 1993. *Health Status and Health Policy: Allocating Resources to Health Care*, New York, Oxford University Press.

Rennie, D., 1995. "Reporting randomized controlled trials: an experiment and a call for responses from readers," *JAMA*, Vol. 273, pp. 1054–1055.

Richardson, W.S., and Detsky, A.S., for the Evidence-Based Medicine Working Group, 1995a. "Users' guides to the medical literature: VII. How to use a clinical decision analysis. A. Are the results of the study valid?" *JAMA*, Vol. 273, pp. 1292–1295.

Richardson, W.S., and Detsky, A.S., for the Evidence-Based Medicine Working Group, 1995b. "Users' guides to the medical literature: VII. How to use a clinical decision analysis. B. What are the results and will they help me in caring for my patients?" *JAMA*, Vol. 273, pp. 1610–1613.

Roper, W.L., Winkenwerder, W., Hackbarth, G.M., et al., 1988. "Effectiveness in health care: an initiative to evaluate and improve medical practice," *New England Journal of Medicine*, Vol. 319, pp. 1197–1202.

Sloan, F., ed., 1995. *Valuing Health Care: Costs, Benefits, and Effectiveness of Pharmaceuticals and Other Medical Technologies*, New York, Cambridge University Press.

Sox, H.C., ed., 1990. *Common Diagnostic Tests: Use and Interpretation*, 2nd ed., Philadelphia, PA, American College of Physicians.

Stewart, A.L., and Ware, J.E., Jr., eds., 1992. *Measuring Functioning and Well-Being*, Durham, NC, Duke University Press.

Stuart, M.E., and Handley, M.A., n.d. *An Evidence-Based Approach to Changing Clinical Practice*, Seattle, WA, Group Health Cooperative of Puget Sound.

Task Force on Principles for Economic Analysis of Health Care Technology, 1995. "Economic analysis of health care technology: a report on principles," *Annals of Internal Medicine*, Vol. 122, pp. 61–70.

U.S. Food and Drug Administration, Center for Drug Evaluation and Research, 1988. *Guideline for the Format and Content of the Clinical and Statistical Sections of New Drug Applications*, Rockville, MD.

U.S. General Services Administration, 1991. *Code of Federal Regulations*, Subchapter D, "Drugs for human use," Title 21, Parts 300–499, Washington, DC, April 1.

Warner, K.E., and Luce, B.R., 1982. *Cost-Benefit and Cost-Effectiveness Analysis in Health Care: Principles, Practice, and Potential*, Ann Arbor, MI, Health Administration Press.

Chapter Four

USING THE RESULTS OF TECHNOLOGY ASSESSMENT

Technology assessment appears to be well established in the organizations interviewed for study, thus supporting the view that a strong private-sector demand exists for TA. However, how widely TA has diffused into the managed care, hospital, or other sectors of the health care system is not known, nor is the likelihood of how far that diffusion will extend in the next five years. Moreover, whether the organizations that have made a commitment to TA today will be among the economic winners or losers in tomorrow's competitive health-care marketplace is unknown.

What *is* known is that the National Committee on Quality Assurance's inclusion, in early 1995, of a TA requirement for accreditation of health maintenance organizations guarantees the further diffusion of TA in managed care. And, given that hospitals will face greater incentives to manage medical technology in a cost-effective way in the immediate future, the incentives to conduct TAs in that sector can also be expected to increase.

For physicians, increased TA can be expected by some medical specialties, such as radiology (Fryback, 1995), that have a well-established tradition of evaluating the economic implications of technologies. But, in general, how changing patterns of physician practice and organization will affect physician incentives to use TA is not readily apparent. Specialty societies may place greater emphasis on clinical practice guidelines than on TA, because guidelines are more immediately and directly related to medical practice.

The emergence of a robust TA capability, in concert with the widespread development of clinical practice guidelines and the creation of applied health services research units, should be recognized as representing a new model for translating the results of medical research into scientifically based clinical practice. To overstate for the sake of argument: The older model assumed that medical research reported in the peer-reviewed literature was read and synthesized by the individual physician in his or her office or was effectively summarized in continuing medical education (CME) courses, and that individual physicians modified their practice accordingly. The older model, in short, held that good information led to behavioral change.

However, researchers, including those who assess medical technologies, often overestimate the effect that good scientific research, clinical-trials results, practice guidelines, and TAs have on physician behavior and on the costs and quality of care. The behavioral literature suggests that it is difficult to change practices by relying on information alone.

The new model is predicated on the assumption that a systematic and comprehensive evaluation of the science underlying medical practice is a multi-step process and requires a deliberately organized effort that is well beyond the capabilities of the busy physician in his or her office or most CME programs. The results reported in this study suggest strongly that this assumption has a sound foundation in practice in the private sector of medicine.

Moreover, TA organizations need to see themselves as institutions engaged in the translation of medical science into validated clinical knowledge, in concert with other evaluative efforts, such as clinical practice guidelines and health services research. This recognition appears to be taking hold, as the preceding chapters indicate. Behavioral change is possible when TA information is reinforced by feedback and educational mechanisms, in settings where the economic incentives to use information are favorable. Systems that deal with all aspects of generating and using the results of TAs are beginning to be developed. This chapter documents some of these systems for coverage decisionmaking, handling terminal illness, providing feedback to member services, and managing technology use, as well as the emergent infrastructure of technology assessment.

COVERAGE DECISIONMAKING

The emergence of TA subscription services strongly suggests that assessments have utility. BCBSA and ECRI, for example, depend primarily on the willingness of new and continuing subscribers to *pay* for their services. Although BCBSA and ECRI do little *monitoring* of actual use, it appears that TA subscription services (1) offer a point of reference for an organization conducting its own TA and (2) are inputs to organizational decisions about coverage.

An example of the use of subscription services is provided by CIGNA, one of the nation's largest managed care organizations, with 3.3 million members in approximately 45 health plans. In the Hartford home office, CIGNA has a centralized TA function managed by one full-time professional who reports to the National Medical Director. CIGNA does not conduct TAs itself, but subscribes to the BCBSA Technology Evaluation Service and attends meetings of the Blue Cross Medical Advisory Panel. When CIGNA receives an assessment from BCBSA, it reviews the TA with its own Technology Assessment and Case Review Council of 7–8 members, who are drawn from the medical directors of the plans. This council considers the political, insurance, benefit, legal, and ethical issues associated with an assessment, then converts the BCBSA assessment to a CIGNA policy. In addition, CIGNA contracts with four medical schools—Columbia University, Emory University, University of California at San Diego, and the University of Chicago—to review cases involving individual patients.

FLEXIBILITY FOR HANDLING TERMINAL ILLNESS

Coverage decisionmaking has typically been binary: Either a procedure or technology is approved or it is not. If not approved, a request by a physician or patient for payment for a procedure is denied. This rigidity has created problems when the effectiveness of a procedure has not been established but the patient has a terminal illness and the procedure is believed by experts to be the "best available" treatment. In particular, the use of high-dose chemotherapy with autologous bone marrow transplantation for the treatment of breast cancer has been the focus of substantial controversy, including costly litigation.

Aetna has responded to the complexities of high-visibility terminal-illness cases involving high-technology, high-risk, and high-cost medical procedures by stimulating the creation of the Medical Care Ombudsman Program (MCOP), an independent organization, to review the appropriateness of care for individual terminal patients. Aetna made an initial policy decision that a procedure being evaluated in a Phase III[1] National Cancer Institute clinical trial meet a prima facie test of "substantial promise" of effectiveness, a term of art but a decidedly weaker one than the claim that "effectiveness has been established."

When cases arise in which patient and physician wish to have such a procedure and request authorization and payment for it, but the health plan medical director questions the procedure's appropriateness on the grounds that it has not been shown to be effective, Aetna does not automatically deny coverage as it would have previously. It now refers such cases to the MCOP of the Medical Care Management Corporation in Bethesda, Maryland.

The MCOP has established, and maintains a roster of, nationally prominent, board-certified experts, most of whom are oncologists. These experts are available to review specific cases as they occur. Typically, a review involves three experts, each of whom independently examines the patient's medical record and makes a recommendation about the appropriateness of the specific procedure for the individual patient. If one expert recommends that treatment is appropriate for the patient, Aetna covers the procedure for that patient. If all three experts recommend against treatment, they agree in advance to go to court, if necessary, and defend their judgment.

The merits of this approach are that the patient and the treating physician receive the benefit of a patient-specific expert review of appropriateness, the coverage determination is based on the judgments of nationally recognized experts, and the insurer has a basis for a decision that minimizes its legal liability. MCOP now has over 100 corporate clients, and has processed more than 2,500 cases that involve new procedures about which substantial scientific uncer-

---

[1]In Phase I trials, safety and pharmacological profiling in humans is tested; Phase II trials involve initial testing of effectiveness in humans; and Phase III trials involve extensive clinical trials of effectiveness in humans.

tainty exists and for which evidence-based TAs have yet to provide a clear indication of effectiveness.   This institutional response introduces flexibility in a heretofore-rigid coverage-decision process.

MEMBER SERVICE FEEDBACK

Many uses of TAs go beyond what can be gained from subscription services, which involve minimal feedback to the TA performer about actual use. An example of increasing feedback to members is provided by University HealthSystem Consortium (UHC), which has been engaged in the systematic production of TAs since 1992. In the past 2–3 years, it has developed various mechanisms for increasing the use of TA among its members.

One mechanism has been a benchmarking project conducted with Sun Health Systems. The project surveyed 400 hospitals (9 in the Sun system, all of the member hospitals of UHC, and some non-UHC, non-Sun hospitals) to obtain baseline data about the nature and extent of TA activity. Of the 93 respondents, about three-quarters were single hospitals and the rest were equally divided between multi-hospital systems and integrated delivery systems. Only 5 percent of the hospitals had a single individual who was solely responsible for technology assessment. Almost one-half of the respondents reported that responsibility for the evaluation of capital equipment (45 percent) and clinical services (55 percent) resided in one individual, as distinct from a group or formal committee. However, in over 90 percent of the responses, evaluation of pharmaceuticals was the responsibility of a formal committee. The use of standard formats for supporting data ranged from a low of 9 percent in the assessment of information systems to 40 percent for evaluation of drugs. In generating such data, basic as they are, UHC has sought to highlight for its members the limited systematic attention being given to technology assessment and to encourage greater effort (Sun Health Alliance, 1995).

A second UHC effort attempted to help member organizations to plan and implement a strategy "to limit and/or reduce expenditures" for radiopaque contrast agents. A report issued in January 1995 (UHC, 1995) summarized a 1993 assessment on "low osmolality contrast media" (LOCM), which, in turn, had updated a 1991 assessment. The 1993 TA recommended that formal guidelines be developed for use of LOCM, that the American College of Radiology and American College of Cardiology guidelines on this topic be used as a starting point, that a compliance-oversight mechanism be established, and that guidelines be continuously reevaluated and revised. In addition, the 1995 report documented recent LOCM successes at two institutions—the University Medical Center, Tucson, and the University of Pittsburgh Medical Center—and added descriptive abstracts of the experience of the University of North Carolina Hospitals and the Robert Wood Johnson University Hospital in New Jersey. These reports indicated the annual savings to each hospital (or system) from implementing LOCM protocols and guidelines.

Finally, UHC hosted an educational conference in early October 1995 on stereotactic radiosurgery, for which two devices are on the market: one costing $1.5 million and the other, $3 million. There is little scientific literature evaluating the devices' clinical effectiveness and cost-effectiveness relative to each other. In fact, UHC identified 16 member hospitals that had been prepared to buy the more expensive device. They were not aware that the other machine was available. The conference, which brought together clinicians, administrators, CEOs, and Chief Financial Officers, successfully highlighted the unsupported claims of the expensive device and led to a clinical trial by the manufacturer of that system.

MANAGEMENT OF TECHNOLOGY USE

Another use of TA is to provide options for those insurers, managed care organizations, and health plans that wish for, or must respond to, innovation, medical practice, and technology management other than by simple approval or denial of coverage of a technology or procedure. Blue Cross Blue Shield of Oregon illustrates uses of TA to aid in a more orderly introduction of medical technology than was characteristic under fee-for-service medicine as recently as five years ago.

In the early 1990s, BCBSA decided to participate with the National Cancer Institute in clinical trials of high-dose chemotherapy with the support of autologous bone marrow transplantation (ABMT) for the treatment of breast cancer. A set of Blue Cross plans agreed to finance the patient-care portion for their beneficiaries with breast cancer if patients were willing to enroll in an NCI randomized clinical trial (RCT) that included ABMT.

Although the overall experience with this initiative has been disappointing, given that many women have refused to be randomized and that patient accrual was slow, it has been very satisfactory for Blue Cross Blue Shield of Oregon. The Medicare Director of Oregon BCBS found that the ABMT clinical-trial option freed him from the tyranny of a Yes/No (approve/deny) coverage decision. It allowed him to say to a physician that it was not known whether the treatment was effective but that the option for that treatment was available if the patient would enroll in a clinical trial. In three years of experience with approximately 50 subscribers, BCBS of Oregon has met all but one of the subscribers' concerns: Most women were enrolled in an RCT, some were turned down for the procedure, and a few (e.g., three men) who were not eligible for an RCT had the ABMT service paid for in a non-RCT study.

An extension of this development is that Oregon BCBS is beginning to take the initiative in identifying those medical centers most qualified to conduct clinical trials of new procedures and to which it will direct beneficiaries. In the future, this data will allow BCBS of Oregon to provide better information about clinical effectiveness than would be obtained if it simply relied on the recommendations of enthusiasts for a procedure. One such new procedure for this initiative is magnetic resonance angiography (MRA), a noninvasive procedure for the diagnosis of cerebral vascular disease in at-risk patients. It has the prospect of replacing conventional angiography, an invasive diagnostic procedure with a number of risks. MRA is basically a software add-on to an already-installed magnetic resonance imaging (MRI) machine. Compared with the multimillion-dollar cost of the MRI machine, which has already been absorbed, the add-on cost of several hundred thousand dollars for MRA is modest. The advent of MRA, however, also opens the possibility of using the technique to screen asymptomatic patients, who are usually diagnosed by ultrasound. Screening complicates the potential cost substantially, raising again the issue of duplicate and overlapping tests (ultrasound and MRA).

BCBS of Oregon is paying for the procedure in Bend, Oregon, where high-quality images are being obtained with a third-generation MRA program; first-generation images are not being reimbursed. The literature at this time is not helpful, according to Dr. John Santa, the BCBS of Oregon Medical Director: "It [the literature] says that MRA is coming, it's not quite here, yet it will be here soon" (personal interview, 1995). Consequently, BCBS of Oregon surveyed neurologists, neurosurgeons, and vascular surgeons and asked two questions: (1) "If MRA is done, are you using the images to make treatment decisions?" and (2) "Has MRA replaced conventional angiography?" The answers were: First, in the centers approved by BCBS of Oregon for this diagnostic procedure, MRA images are being used to make treatment decisions. Second, MRA has clearly replaced conventional angiography in these centers.

Technical competition among imaging modalities is changing the situation still further. Sufficiently good images of the carotid artery are now being obtained with ultrasound (US), a competing modality, so that some surgeons are proceeding to operate on the basis of the US image alone—without using either conventional angiography or MRA.

Radiologists were also surveyed for data showing that MRA has replaced conventional angiography. They confirmed that MRA has replaced angiography in approved demonstration sites. Dr. Santa reports one radiologist as saying: "This is an interesting exercise. It lets me tell my colleagues that we can't get by just by showing them the images. We have to have data that show the effect" (personal interview, 1995).

Dr. Santa expressed a more general interest in technology "roll out" strategies, which involve designating regional centers for exclusive reimbursement in the initial stage of a new technology. Those centers would be required to develop protocols for use and would then be asked to teach others how to provide treatment using the protocols. As the technology diffused beyond the initially designated centers, adherence to protocols would become a criterion for reimbursement.

Oregon BCBS has implemented a similar strategy for sleep-disorder studies, is doing so for MRA and brachytherapy for prostate cancer, and is considering such a strategy for pallidotomy, minimally invasive surgery, and lung-reduction surgery. The intent is to avoid episodes such as the oncologists' advocacy of ABMT and the general surgeons' advocacy of laparoscope cholesystectomy, both of which diffused widely before they were evaluated adequately.

THE EMERGENT INFRASTRUCTURE

Several respondents in this study commented that "the science of application had lagged the science of discovery," that is, the investment in research, including TA, had not been accompanied by an appropriate investment in examining how such research was used. They argued that an applied clinical or health-services-research capability was needed.

As the *application* of TA, practice guidelines, and health services research in general advances, institutional channels of communication and hierarchies of decisionmaking are being established that link the generators, synthesizers, and users of clinical science—medical research, technology assessment, and practice guidelines—in new and tighter relationships. One important development in this respect is the emergence of a decentralized TA performer capability, as indicated in Chapter Two. It is important to recognize that this robust *performer capability* is also creating a more decentralized *user capability*. These increasingly decentralized users might be regarded as an increased number of *receptor sites*, which can only facilitate communication from TA performers to TA users. Greater demand for TA, a decentralized TA performer capability, an enhanced concern for evidence-based clinical practice, and an increasingly sophisticated set of TA users are factors that suggest that the use of TA is likely to increase in the future.

The model, or strategy, of TA implementation should, at a minimum, be at least as sophisticated as the strategies that drug companies have used in the past for influencing the prescribing behavior of individual, office-based physicians. Among other things, they should recognize the importance of the following: the demand for TA as a critical factor in its eventual use; the existence of a TA capability that can translate existing scientific information into usable form; the establishment and maintenance of communication channels from TA producers to prospective users; the transmission of assessments through those channels; attention to the incentives governing the use of TA at the receptor sites for the information, comparing it to current practice, and modifying behavior as appropriate; the accountable reporting of experience to interested parties; and the establishment and maintenance of feedback loops among all elements in the system.

In the face of increased demand for TA and other evaluative activities, it may be appropriate for the federal government to support work on the development and diffusion of strategies to move both TA methodologies and results into operational use.

REFERENCES

Fryback, D.G., ed., 1995. *Introduction to Technology Assessment for Radiologists: Vision Beyond Tomorrow, Vols. 1 and 2*, Milwaukee, WI, GE Medical Systems—Association of University Radiologists Radiology Research Academic Fellowship (GERRAF) Program.

Sun Health Alliance, in cooperation with University Hospital Consortium, 1995. *Best Practices in Technology Assessment*, A Report to the Sun Health Alliance and the University Hospital Consortium from the Technology Assessment Benchmarking Team, Oak Brook, IL, April.

University HealthService Consortium, Clinical Practice Advancement Center, 1995. *Technology Assessment Implementation Case Study: Radiopaque Contrast Media*, Oak Brook, IL, January.

Chapter Five

IMPLICATIONS FOR PUBLIC-PRIVATE RELATIONSHIPS

The preceding chapters discuss technology assessment in the private health care sector, focusing on TA in managed care organizations— not on government TA activity, which has been the focus of much of the literature on TA. Here, we step back and ask two questions:

- What major conclusions flow from this analysis?

- What are the implications of these conclusions for relations between public- and private-sector TA and for the role of the federal government in technology assessment?

THE DEMAND FOR TA

The demand for TA in the private sector of the U.S. health care system appears to be strong and, as suggested by this report, to have increased substantially in recent years. However, no precise baseline data have been collected from which to measure this demand, and no quantitative estimates of its magnitude have been put forward. Although this demand has sometimes focused explicitly on technology assessment, more often the demand for TA is embedded in the search for evaluative tools that support cost containment, and quality measurement and improvement.

The primary source of this increased demand for evaluative services has been the purchasers of health care, especially large corporations. Managed care health organizations are the second major source. They are responding both to purchasers and to what they see as their strategic needs and opportunities in the marketplace.

The primary implication of this increased private-sector TA is that an opportunity exists for public and private sectors to reinforce each other in constructive ways. The call for rigorous evaluation of health care cost and quality, whether through technology assessment or other evaluative approaches, is shared by organizations in both sectors.

Another major implication of the increased private-sector demand for TA is that the federal government, in its capacity as a major *purchaser* of health care services, should act comparably to the private sector. The argument for an aggressive (i.e., competent and effective) federal government purchaser of health care services is sound at both conceptual and practical levels: Medicare and Medicaid expenditures in federal and state government spending are significant, and efforts are currently being promoted to increase the reliance on managed care in both programs. Therefore, the federal government should strengthen its capability to assess the value of services provided by those programs, both for individual beneficiaries and for populations of patients.

For the federal government to act more aggressively as a prudent buyer of health services, which includes a more aggressive use of TA, poses political challenges that should be clearly understood. The prudent-buyer role of the government often has been limited by the frequent opposition of beneficiaries, providers, and suppliers to such a role. The response to these groups? In its quest for value for health care expenditures, the government should be no less effective a purchaser of health care than purchasers in the private sector.

However, to increase its capability as a purchaser, the federal government does not need to create a large, centralized TA organization. It may acquire some of its assessments by contracting with the private sector, as CHAMPUS has done with Blue Cross Blue Shield Association and as HCFA has done with ECRI. Nonetheless, it would be prudent for the government to maintain TA competence to ensure a TA-contract-management capability, to stay abreast of methodological developments in the field, to contribute to assessment-related research, and to avoid complete dependence on the private sector.

THE PERFORMERS OF TECHNOLOGY ASSESSMENT

The second conclusion pertains to the *performers* of TA in the United States. The aspirations for the strong national TA entity envisioned in the 1970s and 1980s, which encompassed research related to medical technology and its evaluation, coverage advice to HCFA, and TA leadership for the entire U.S. health care system, have not materialized. Instead, a distributed set of TA performers has emerged in the private health care sector in the past several years. Centralized in some aspects and decentralized in others, this distributed "system" encompasses a robust analytical capability that did not exist a decade ago. The federal government is today only one player in technology assessment, and not the dominant one, and is in a relatively weak position to exert leadership along the lines envisioned in the 1980s. The modest volume of output of OHTA, for example, exerts little leverage on the actions of others.

What are the implications of these organizational developments? One implication is that the public-private *division of labor* in technology assessment needs to be reconsidered. A benefit of the distributed private TA system is that both the number and range of those TAs performed are greater than in a centralized system, reflecting both greater expression of demand and more-extensive TA performer responses. Moreover, the market will tend to equilibrate TA performers and users on the number of assessments required, as well as among competing services in assigning cost-quality or price-quality trade-offs.

However, the *standards* set by the market for the conduct of TA will be implicit: the product of the incentives driving demand for assessments and the prevailing views about acceptable methodology. This potentially arbitrary conjunction suggests a possible role for the federal government in supporting explicit standards of methodologic rigor, either by regulating requirements or by highlighting methodologic rigor in a sustained and visible way. Short of establishing regulatory authority comparable to that of the FDA, the means for effectively requiring such rigor are far from clear. However, methodological research offers a legitimate and acceptable way for the federal government to assist in setting and maintaining standards for performing technology assessment. Less driven by market forces, the government is in a much better position than the private sector to strengthen current methodologies—e.g., by generating more primary data, strengthening weak methods, increasing the use of strong methods, and training TA researchers— and to address methodological challenges that arise as the field continues to develop.

More generally, the above paragraphs suggest that one role for the federal government is the support of *TA-related research*. The value of research results cannot be captured solely by the perfomer of research. For this reason, the private sector has an incentive to under-invest in the socially optimal level of research, including TA-related research. Only the government can respond to the need for research. Ironically, although the National Center for Health Care Technology (1978–1982) was established legislatively to support research, it met its end largely because a delegation of PHS administrative authority required it to support Medicare coverage decisionmaking. A consequence of its demise was that little TA-related research has been supported by the federal government in the past two decades. It may now be appropriate to review the need for such research.

A different implication deals with the matter of *multiple studies*. At present, many TA users obtain the services of more than one TA performer, but few users obtain *all* available services, behavior that allows a balance to be struck between useful redundancy and unnecessary duplication. Although centralization of TA has often been justified by the need to eliminate duplication, too little attention has been given to the value of redundancy or of overlapping and multiple studies. It is seldom the case that a single study, clinical trial, or assessment is definitive for clinical effectiveness or cost-effectiveness. Redundancy among competing TA services, therefore, allows for a validation process to occur by which the assessments of one TA organization are compared with those of another.

Recognizing the value of multiple studies forces the issue of *coordination* to be reconsidered. It is often assumed that a centralized body is better able to coordinate multiple performers than are multiple organizations in a distributed, market-based system. This argument overlooks the value of redundancy, discussed above, and also ignores the administrative requirements of coordination. Administrative resources—time, money, and personnel—are always scarce, and centralized coordination is vulnerable to bottlenecks or queuing at all stages of the TA process—priority-setting, conducting assessments, and reporting results.

By contrast, a distributed TA system of many assessment organizations manages to coordinate both TA producers and users. On the user side, as mentioned above, many TA users obtain several of the available TA services and, via the low-priced newsletter products, can easily track all relevant TA performers. On the performer side, as the director of one TA program said: "I submit that all quality TA organizations review the work of other TA organizations, e.g., I have collaborative document-sharing with ECRI, AMA, AHA, etc. And I expect my TA authors to always review the TA work of others (e.g., OHTA, AHCPR, ECRI, USP-DI, international, etc.) to continually build on the strengths of existing work" (Karl Matuszewski, interview).

EVIDENCE-BASED TA

Among those organizations interviewed during this research, the dominant characteristic of TA in the private sector in the mid-1990s is the prevalence and strength of the underlying commitment to *evidence-based assessments.* This emphasis on systematically and rigorously assessing clinical effectiveness is clearly new. At one level, it reflects the seriousness with which the evaluation of medical care is now being undertaken—a result of the diffusion of health services research into the financing organization, delivery, and practice of medicine. It also reflects a movement beyond reliance on informal canvassing of expert opinion as a way to establish the science underlying clinical practice. Evidence-based assessment, still in its youth, both broadens and deepens the evaluation of medical technologies in the following ways:

* It is broader than the evaluation of therapeutic *products* (drugs, biologics, and devices) for safety and effectiveness, and includes clinical *procedures.*

* It extends clinical-effectiveness assessments of both products and procedures to ask about their *relative clinical effectiveness,* i.e., how a technology compares with no treatment and with competitive interventions, potentially subjecting "me-too"

products and marginally beneficial procedures to a new level of scrutiny.

• It goes beyond the FDA's narrow evaluation of *pharmaceuticals* for safety and efficacy to the broader assessments by P&T committees of relative clinical effectiveness and cost-effectiveness.

• It connects the concern for *value*, i.e., the relation of resources and outcomes, prospectively to cost-effectiveness analysis (see below).

• It underscores the dependence of the assessment process on *clinical trials* and highlights the *management weaknesses* of many trials in terms of poor design and controls, slow patient accrual, poor quality of data management, and inconclusive results reported in the literature (see below).

This commitment to evidence-based assessments, which characterizes AHCPR's efforts both in TA and clinical practice guidelines, reinforces the need for all parties—public and private—to search for ways to strengthen this commitment whenever possible.

How might such strengthening be done? A more aggressive use of TA by the federal government as a major purchaser of services has been suggested above, as has a sustained TA-related research effort, especially one focused on methodological issues. Other approaches that might be considered include searching for ways to make cost-effectiveness analysis more useful as a tool in operational settings and in improving the quality of clinical trials.

Cost-Effectiveness Analysis

Although it has been discussed for more than a decade, the actual use of *cost-effectiveness analysis* in technology assessment has been quite limited. However, as the demand for more-rigorous evaluation of clinical effectiveness has increased, so too has the demand for CEA. One factor limiting the use of CEA has been that its proponents have been mainly academics; there has not been a widespread user community among those in nonacademic settings, which may imply a need for training efforts. More significant, the problems of applying CEA in operational settings, especially those stemming from the limitations of data, deserve systematic attention, perhaps through conferences that bring academics and users together on a regular basis.

Finally, the philosophic issue of whether a societal, community, or even narrower perspective should inform CEA in the competitive marketplace requires more-than-passing acknowledgment. If market incentives drive TA users to adopt a narrow perspective on costs—limiting their analytic concerns to the likely effect of a given technology on health plan premiums or hospital revenues, their competitive position in the local health market, their capacity to attract physicians, etc.—the utility of CEA in a distributed TA system will be limited. Consciousness-raising about CEA has occurred, and tentative steps toward application are being taken. But substantially greater public- and private-sector cooperation can help to clarify both the methodological and philosophical issues of *application* in operational settings.

Clinical Trials

Clinical trials are essential to technology assessments. Evidence-based TAs always involve a literature review, usually the compilation of evidence tables, sometimes meta-analyses, and often a grading of the studies being examined. In such reviews, the clinical-trials literature frequently receives very low marks on quality. As a result, the distributed TA performers who depend on this literature are increasingly being made aware of its shortcomings.

However, the knowledge that these sophisticated users of the clinical-trials literature have acquired has not yet been transmitted back to the sponsors and performers of trials. Effective feedback loops between the users and the generators of the literature apparently do not exist. Nor are there mechanisms for purchasers of or payers for health care to indicate their priorities for clinical trials, because these priorities are determined largely by academic researchers.

An *institutional disconnect* exists between those payers who wish to know what procedures are clinically effective and the academics who generate the clinical-trials literature. One implication of this disconnect for public-private cooperation is that a series of conferences, workshops, or symposia might be organized to examine the issues associated with the relationship between clinical trials and the effectiveness of new procedures flowing into clinical practice. Such an initiative would involve NIH, FDA, AHCPR, and HCFA, as well as pharmaceutical and medical device firms, academic researchers, and purchasers of and payers for care.

More generally, both public- and private-sector organizations should commit themselves to increasing the proportion of new technologies and procedures subjected to rigorous TA analysis until the *expectation* of such evaluation is shared by all parties, including those bringing new products and procedures to the market, and until those expectations are *embedded in operational policies and procedures*. This commitment is necessary for ensuring that the beachhead of evidence-based assessments is secured and is safely beyond political challenge.

TA AND CLINICAL PRACTICE GUIDELINES

Technology assessment and clinical practice guidelines share an orientation to evidence-based assessments and have essentially a common methodology, although the amount of data available to each may differ. A major factor limiting TAs is the inadequacy of data at the time that a new technology is introduced and when advocates for its use command the relevant "expertise" and press for a favorable coverage decision. The development of guidelines is less likely to be hampered by data limitations in the same way, because the subjects for guidelines are typically procedures, clinical conditions, or disease states for which a good deal of clinical experience exists. But the relative data needs of TA and guidelines deserve attention in an integrated way, as does the search for creative means of data acquisition to serve the ends of each. TAs and guidelines also differ with respect to their focus: TAs deal with specific technologies or procedures, which guidelines may also; but the latter tend to address the management of a clinical condition or disease state. In addition, TAs support coverage decisions in the main; guidelines are oriented to modifying physician behavior.

Although some TA advocates view clinical practice guidelines as a special form of TA, guidelines developers may or may not be aware of TA as they do their work. Moreover, federal government programs have often reified distinctions between TA and related evaluative efforts, such as clinical practice guidelines. As a result, differences are emphasized and commonalities receive less attention.

Importantly at present, the relationship between TA and guidelines is being clarified in private-sector operational settings in ways that simply ignore doctrinal arguments at the conceptual level. The primary implication for public-private cooperation is that the further development of each activity should be coordinated, if not integrated, in the interest of promoting a deeper understanding of differences and commonalities, furthering evidence-based assessment of medical interventions, and advancing concern for the value of health services delivered.

ENCOURAGING THE USE OF TA

As of the mid-1990s, technology assessment has developed to the point where the primary challenge of the next decade is to encourage its widespread diffusion and to develop the strategies and tools of practical application in operational settings. Such diffusion should be directed toward increasing the value of delivered health services by bringing costs under control and into relation with quality.

How should we think about encouraging the uses of TA?

First, encouraging wider use of TA cannot be predicated on the assumption that a good assessment reported in the literature is sufficient to ensure its adoption. A more sophisticated model of information flow and behavior change needs to include attention to the message and its quality, to the source of the message, to the channels of reaching prospective users, to the receptivity of users to the message, and to modification of both TA message content and processes as a result of feedback from users.

Second, meeting this challenge of wider application is made easier by the growth of a physician-based analytic capability committed to evidence-based assessment of new technologies and procedures, and to clinical practice guidelines. It is important to recognize that a corollary of the emergence of a robust, distributed TA *performer* capability is the parallel emergence of a larger number of physicians and other clinicians who are grappling with the implications of TAs and practice guidelines. Thus, a highly decentralized set of *receptor sites* for TA results is coming into being within the physician community. Communication from TA performers is made easier when there are TA users to receive the message.

Third, it should be recognized that the decentralization of TA to multiple performers and users is likely to facilitate physician buy-in to the results of assessments by reducing the remoteness of clinicians from the group conducting the assessment. Assessments done by an organization with which a physician is affiliated, such as a regional or local health plan, are more likely to capture the doctor's attention and have greater face validity than the TAs of a centralized body.

Fourth, TAs should be used consistently as inputs to coverage decisions, even though factors other than evidence-based assessments inevitably enter into, and may determine, the outcome of such decisions.

Fifth, TAs should be used to benchmark best practice and to provide feedback to users through educational conferences and other means.

Sixth, TAs should be used as feedback to the design and sponsorship of clinical trials and to priority-setting for such trials.

Seventh, TAs should also be used to introduce greater flexibility of response to the emergence of new technologies and procedures. Examples of flexible response include using enrollment in clinical trials as a way of dealing with promising but unproved, high-visibility procedures for treating terminally ill patients; using independent third-party evaluation of the appropriateness of an experimental procedure for a specific patient, especially when procedures treat terminally ill patients; and use of TA to promote rational "roll out" of new technologies in patterns of protocol-based, data-driven, controlled diffusion.

Eighth, TAs should be used to reinforce the development and use of evidence-based clinical practice guidelines and to train the next generation of physicians in the meaning and implications of evidence-based medicine.

THE ROLE OF THE FEDERAL GOVERNMENT

Given the vigorous private-sector TA capability, what is the TA role for the federal government? One thing is clear: A federal government leadership role of the kind envisioned in the 1970s and 1980s has very little support. The demise of health-care-reform legislation in 1994 and the current composition of Congress make such a role infeasible. Instead, the possibilities of public-private *cooperation*—which includes coordination, collaboration, contracting, and the production of collective, or public, goods—must be pursued.

Coordination. Is the current informal coordination among public and private TA performers adequate? Although centralized coordination remains the ideal in the minds of a number of individuals, a substantial amount of coordination now takes place informally, with every TA organization basically keeping book on every other TA organization. Information flows easily, if not freely, in this distributed TA system. This decentralized and informal coordination among TA performers may be as effective or efficient as that of centralized coordination. It is not demonstrably worse.

Collaboration is another form of cooperation that involves some mutual contribution of resources to a common effort. Although attractive in principle, collaboration is difficult to organize in practice: Public bodies may have private advisory committees but may not delegate decisionmaking to such bodies, except by statute; private entities may have public liaison representatives, but public officials may not serve in official capacities in such organizations; and the commingling of public and private resources is not readily sanctioned.

"Soft" collaboration between the government and the private sector regarding TA may occur, however, through informal coordination and formal contracting. It may be the most effective way to help the government fulfill its obligations as a value-oriented purchaser of health care, on the premise that it should be as effective a purchaser as the private sector. Although enrolling more Medicare beneficiaries in managed care will limit HCFA's role in defining the benefit package, a continued fiduciary role remains for Medicare to ensure that effective health care is purchased for these beneficiaries, especially as smaller health plans assume greater responsibility for providing health care services. Examples of soft collaboration include agreement on the criteria for reporting the results of TAs, clinical trials, and effectiveness research, and other efforts to strengthen the methodological foundation of these activities.

Contracting may be seen as a form of public-private cooperation. It is the approach now being taken by CHAMPUS, which contracts with BCBSA for TA services, and by HCFA, which contracts with ECRI. For contract management to be effective, however, it is necessary to retain a technical capability within the government in order to avoid undue reliance on the private sector.

Finally, the *production of public goods* argues for cooperation when the benefits of an activity are available to all and cannot be captured by the party generating the benefits. In such situations, the private sector faces economic incentives that will cause it to invest in that activity at a level below what is socially optimal. Research, especially on analytical methodologies, is this kind of public good and defines a role for the federal government. Such research ought to include the further development of TA methodologies, especially the methodologies of application, both for analytic and standard-setting purposes. Research defined by the federal government role would encompass the conduct of clinical trials, priority-setting for such trials, cost-effectiveness analysis, increased evaluation of new drugs by managed care organizations, and the implications of such special topics as the revolution in genetics and molecular biology and appropriate TA responses to treatments for terminal illness.